Emotional Labour in Health Care

Do nurses still care? In today's inflexible, fast-paced and more accountable workplace where biomedical and clinical models dominate health care practice, is there room for emotional labour?

Based on original empirical research, this book delves into the personal accounts of nurses' emotional expressions and experiences as they emerge from everyday nursing practice, and illustrates how their emotional labour is adapting in response to a constantly changing work environment.

The book begins by re-examining Arlie Hochschild's sociological notion of emotional labour, and combines it with Margaret Archer's understanding of emotion and the inner dialogue. In an exploration of the nature of emotional labour, its historical and political context, and providing an original but easily recognisable typology, Catherine Theodosius emphasises that it is emotion – complex, messy and opaque – that drives emotional labour within health care. She suggests that, rather than being marginalised, emotional labour in nursing is frequently found in places that are often hidden or unrecognised. By understanding emotion itself, which is fundamentally interactive and communicative, she argues that emotional labour is intrinsically linked to personal and social identity. The suggestion is made that the nursing profession has a responsibility to include emotional labour within personal and professional development strategies to ensure the care needs of the vulnerable are met.

This innovative volume will be of interest to nursing, health care and sociology students, researchers and professionals.

Catherine Theodosius recently completed an ESRC postdoctoral fellowship at the University of Essex and is a Lecturer in Adult Nursing at University Campus Suffolk.

Critical Studies in Health and Society
Series Editors
Simon J. Williams and Gillian Bendelow

This major new international book series takes a critical look at health in a rapidly changing social world. The series includes theoretically sophisticated and empirically informed contributions on cutting-edge issues from leading figures within the sociology of health and allied disciplines and domains. Other titles in the series include:

Contesting Psychiatry
Social movements in mental health
Nick Crossley

Men and their Health
Masculinity, social inequality and health
Alan Dolan

Lifestyle in Medicine
Gary Easthope and Emily Hansen

Medial Sociology and Old Age
Towards a sociology of health in later life
Paul Higgs and Ian Rees Jones

Written in a lively, accessible and engaging style, with many thought-provoking insights, the series will cater to a truly interdisciplinary audience of researchers, professionals, practitioners and policy makers with an interest in health and social change.

Those interested in submitting proposals for single or co-authored, edited or co-edited volumes should contact the series editors, Simon J. Williams (s.j.williams@warwick.ac.uk) and Gillian Bendelow (g.a.bendelow@sussex.ac.uk).

Emotional Labour in Health Care

The unmanaged heart of nursing

Catherine Theodosius

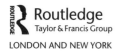

Routledge
Taylor & Francis Group

LONDON AND NEW YORK

First published 2008
by Routledge
2 Park Square, Milton Park, Abingdon, Oxon OX14 4RN

Simultaneously published in the USA and Canada
by Routledge
270 Madison Avenue, New York, NY 10016

Routledge is an imprint of the Taylor & Francis Group, an informa business

Text © 2008 Catherine Theodosius
Illustrations © 2008 Jo Rice

Typeset in Sabon by
Keystroke, 28 High Street, Tettenhall, Wolverhampton
Printed and bound in Great Britain by
CPI Antony Rowe, Chippenham, Wilts

British Library Cataloguing in Publication Data
A catalogue record for this book is available from the British Library

Library of Congress Cataloging in Publication Data
Theodosius, Catherine.
Emotional labour in health care : the unmanaged heart of nursing / Catherine Theodosius.
p. ; cm. – (Critical studies in health and society)
1. Nursing–Psychological aspects. 2. Nurse and patient. 3. Emotions.
I. Title. II. Series.
[DNLM: 1. Nurses–psychology. 2. Emotions. 3. Nursing Care–psychology.
WY 87 T389e 2008]
RT86.T45 2008
610.73–dc22
2007051467

ISBN 10: 0–415–40953–5 (hbk)
ISBN 10: 0–415–40954–3 (pbk)
ISBN 10: 0–203–89495–2 (ebk)

ISBN 13: 978–0–415–40953–7 (hbk)
ISBN 13: 978–0–415–40954–4 (pbk)
ISBN 13: 978–0–203–89495–8 (ebk)

In memory of John and Ivy Hudson

Contents

List of illustrations   ix
Table of vignettes   xi
Preface   xiii
Acknowledgements   xv

Introduction: challenging current conceptualisations
of emotional labour   1

PART I
**Understanding emotional labour in nursing: a theoretical
approach**   9

Vignette 1 'Half measures'   11
1   Emotion management and emotional labour: the work
    of Arlie Russell Hochschild   13

Vignette 2 'Alix's dad'   27
2   Emotional labour in health care   29

Vignette 3 'The scrotal drain'   49
3   Emotion and cognition   51

Vignette 4 'The murderer'   65
4   Synthesising Darwin and Freud with interactionist theory   68

Vignette 5 'Maxine's rant'   88
5   Emotion and personal and social identity   90

PART II
Developing emotional labour in nursing: a theoretically informed empirical approach   **115**

    Vignette 6 'An average shift'   *117*
6 The emotional field   120

    Vignette 7 'The complaint'   *142*
7 Therapeutic emotional labour   143

    Vignette 8 'The NG tube'   *158*
8 Instrumental emotional labour   161

    Vignette 9 'Breaking the shame spiral'   *174*
9 Collegial emotional labour   178

    Vignette 10 'The dying lady'   *198*
10 Reflexive emotion management   201

    Bibliography   220
    Index   227

Illustrations

Figures

5.1	Negative feedback in the inner dialogue	109
6.1	Ward B layout	127
9.1	Typology of emotional labour	196

Tables

3.1	Four key differences between the emotional labour of nurses and that of flight attendants	53
5.1	Emotion orders	93
5.2	The inner dialogue	100
7.1	Therapeutic emotional labour	147
8.1	Instrumental emotional labour	163
9.1	Collegial emotional labour	182

Cartoons

Speed-up!	23
Characteristics of emotional labour	30
Emotional juggler	38
Emotion constructionist	52
Cognition ice cream	57
Emotion work	72
Self-deception	75
Empty bed syndrome	79
Sudden panic	85
The concert pianist	95
Caring for the vomiting patient	107
Nursing stories	134
Exchanging confidences	145
Don't worry!	165
Learning clinical skills	166

Communication conduit   179
The handmaiden!   181
The perfect nurse   216
Working together   219

Table of vignettes

Vignette	Nurse	Data source	Designation	Subgroup
1 Half measures	Paris	Interview	F grade	Beta
2 Alix's dad	Amelia	Audio diary and interview	E grade	Seniors
3 The scrotal drain	Catherine	Participant observation diary	D grade	Beta
4 The murderer	Susan	Interview	D grade	Beta → Populars
5 Maxine's rant	Maxine	Audio diary	E grade	Beta
6 An average shift	Paula	Audio diary	E grade	Seniors
7 The complaint	Emily	Audio diary	E grade	Populars
8 The NG tube	Kate	Interview	D grade	Beta → Seniors
9 Breaking the shame spiral	Kate	Audio diary	D grade	Beta → Seniors
10 The dying lady	Kate	Interview	D grade	Beta → Seniors

Note: At the time of the research, the system of grading nurses in the NHS was as follow:
A and B grades: health care assistant
C grade: starting grade for an enrolled nurse
D grade: starting grade for a qualified registered nurse (junior staff nurse)
E grade: senior staff nurse
F grade: junior sister or charge nurse
G grade: senior sister or charge nurse
H grade: senior manager or clinician

Preface

Since my first introduction to Arlie Russell Hochschild's (1983) *The Managed Heart* as an undergraduate sociology student, I have been fascinated by her notion of emotional labour. To me, she fills that gap in social theory which seems to comment on a society filled with human beings with no heart or soul. For years her work tantalised me with the belief that holism, which is so central to the discipline of nursing, was not entirely incompatible with sociology. As a discipline, nursing is often under-represented, mostly because in taking a biopsychosocial approach it constantly borrows its knowledge from these disciplines. This produces some difficulties, as the application of knowledge that is wholly sociological, psychological or biological will only fit so far into one that is holistic. This has been the challenge of this book. Yet Hochschild, in her approach to emotion and the development of her notion of emotional labour, leads the way. I have merely attempted to make this more explicit in its application to nursing. At the same time, I have also tried to develop the *sociological* concept of emotional labour. My attempt to develop Hochschild's notion of emotional labour for nursing has been one in which I believe the best of sociology is brought together with the best of nursing. Bringing the two together in one book has not been easy. The tentative hope is that this book may be of interest to both sociologists and nurses alike; however, there are some chapters that will inevitably be of more interest to sociologists and some to nurses.

At the heart of this book are the nurses' accounts of their emotions and experiences working on Ward B. The aim of the research was always to examine and observe emotional labour as it took place within a nursing context. Gaining ethical clearance to do so took over a year to negotiate. Any research carried out in health care involves the protection of vulnerable people. Ethical permission from the Local Research Ethics Committee, the nursing research committee, the Nursing Director of the National Health Service (NHS) Trust and the G grade sister on Ward B was granted for all aspects of the empirical data collection. All the nurses who recorded audio diaries and were interviewed consented to do so. In addition, as a qualified, registered nurse I am bound by the Nursing and Midwifery Council's Code of Conduct in which I am called on at all times to protect the confidentiality and anonymity of my patients and to act as their advocate. Throughout the research process and in all resulting publications I have adhered to this Code of Conduct. The empirical research focus is on the role of the nurse and not the patient. However, because the importance of interaction to emotional labour is central to its development, some patients are mentioned in respect to the role of the nurse. As with the nurses, the patient's anonymity is protected by pseudonyms. To ensure that they cannot be identified in any other way, I have also changed some of their medical conditions and social circumstances where these are needed to understand the story.

Because there was only one male nurse working on Ward B, in order to protect his identity the pronoun 'she' is used in respect to 'the nurse' throughout the book. The presence of only one male nurse also meant that it has not been possible to develop any kind of gender analysis; the term 'she' has therefore been used as if it were a generic pronoun, and is not an attempt to disregard the many male nurses in the profession.

Acknowledgements

I am extremely grateful to the Economic and Social Research Council (ESRC) for a PhD award and a postdoctoral fellowship from which the research for this book was undertaken and developed, and particularly to Joan Busfield, Ken Plummer and Mike Roper, who supervised me.

I owe a big debt of thanks to all the nurses on Ward B, who allowed me to work with them and who so generously contributed of their time and selves, granting me an insight into their emotional lives.

An earlier version of some of the ideas in Chapter 4 can be found in *Sociology* 40 (5): 893–910; my thanks to Sage for granting permission to reproduce parts here. I am also very much obliged to University of California Press for permission to quote significant amounts from Hochschild's (1983) *The Managed Heart*, and likewise to Cambridge University Press for large quotations originally published in Archer's (2000) *Being Human*.

I would especially like to thank Joanna Rice, who has produced fantastic illustrations providing a welcome relief to the unrelenting flow of words.

My gratitude to Andrew Saunders whose IT skills helped create Figures 6.1 and 9.1.

I would also like to thank Paul McIntosh, Tim Guymer, Caroline Walker and Lil Wills who between them, not only got me started and kept me going, but also helped me in editing the text and thrashing out a few unwieldy ideas.

To my parents, my love and gratitude.

Introduction

Challenging current conceptualisations of emotional labour

You could say that the modern profession of nursing was born out of a passion for human dignity – not just a sense of a practical job well done, but a serious conviction that what is due to people in situations where they are helpless, and even dying, is time, respect and patience, no less than practical skill . . . Sickness and helplessness are not only matters of bodily incapacity – sickness is also about our picture of ourselves. We are damaged or deprived in respect of what we think and imagine who we are. The self is what is ill or hurt or restricted, not simply a set of bodily functions and processes. Healing is therefore about sustaining and restoring that vulnerable sense of who we are. It is about the service of human dignity. In health care professions, a growing number of people now say that the simply personal and relational skills of healing are squeezed out in training, and seriously undervalued in favour of mechanistic skills. For nurses especially, this is a huge and damaging shift away from that fundamental commitment to human dignity. Are we in danger of creating a culture of health care in which there is no recognition of the professional importance of the personal?

(Archbishop Rowan Williams 2006: 8)

Ward B is a busy acute vascular surgical ward in an NHS Hospital Trust in the UK. It is situated towards the back of the hospital on the second floor. As you enter the ward you find yourself in a dark, dingy, carpeted corridor leading to the nurses' station. The corridor is so dim that the main lights are on even on a sunny August morning. There is no doubt that you are on a hospital ward though, as you pass by the kitchen, the sluice, patients' bathrooms and the sister's office. Then at the end of the corridor as you emerge on to the main ward, light from the windows in the bays bursts through, meeting you with sudden warmth. It is like walking into a bustling, noisy marketplace, only with that all pervading, warm, body odour smell, mixed with disinfectant. There are people everywhere. Blue uniforms, brown uniforms, white coats and suits: nurses, doctors, health care assistants (HCAs), pharmacists, physiotherapists and phlebotomists darting around in a seemingly haphazard way. There are patients in their pyjamas queuing for the bathroom, walking around, sitting in a chair or lying in bed. Buzzers go off incessantly, and the phone – there are two – ringing, ringing, ringing.

> **Maxine:** The phone is the bane of my life. It is always ringing and it is always there and as soon as you hear it ringing, you think, I should answer that; but you are in the middle of something else. And then if you do go to the phone it is a relative; if it's a relative of somebody you are nursing you spend five or ten minutes talking to them. But at the back of your mind you're thinking: 'I've left so and so on the commode'; or, 'I have left so and so half stripped because I was washing them'. So it's this push for time, there never seems to be much time to do the things you want to do. Sometimes I think to myself: 'I didn't give her a toothbrush to do her mouth care' and you think how bad you know you feel in the morning if you haven't brushed your teeth.

The ward seems a mess with linen trolleys and skips everywhere. Mid-morning finds the domestic valiantly trying to dish out tea and coffee to the patients while the cleaner trips over everybody and everything as she mops the floor. There's a phlebotomist with her trolley of bottles going from patient to patient, doctors standing at the desk with patients' notes scattered everywhere, a porter with a rather decrepit old wheelchair looking for a patient wanted down in X-ray and a nurse frantically trying to locate the patient's notes. The patients' lockers are covered with magazines and papers, fruit bowls, sweets and toiletries. There are flowers in all conditions on the patients' tables, lockers and on the windowsill; the carpets are covered in old stains:

> **Maria** [D grade nurse]: This ward is very dirty, it is annoying me. Sometimes I am ashamed. Actually, I think that we should talk to Paris [junior sister] maybe she could change something. Sometimes I am working and I am picking up papers and dressings. And this carpet on surgical ward! My god! Carpet on surgical ward! If I would say to somebody, they couldn't believe me!

The ward is so busy you can stand at the nurses' station for twenty minutes before anybody even notices you are there. The nurses are never still for a minute. Even when they are in the middle of one task, somebody else is demanding their attention for something else – a patient wanting a tablet, the doctor wanting an assistant, a relative asking for information, the student not knowing what to do, the HCA informing her of a patient's observations, or the ward clerk with a phone enquiry, or an admission arrives at the same time as a patient is returned from theatre.

> **Maxine:** Sometimes you land on that ward running and you don't stop until you have your break and then you come back from break and you land on the ward running, and you continue to run until suddenly you realise you're sat on the sofa at home, and you have to stop your mind from still running and switch off!

Maria: Yes, you have no time to go to toilet. Yet maybe now when we are saying something like that, somebody can't believe that something like that can happen, but it happens. I was crossing my legs, you know, one pain killer more, then I was on the way to toilet, then phone call about somebody you know, enquire. Then somebody wanted the commode. I remember that I was trying to go to the toilet a few times but it was always something else; a phone call, somebody's bed pump, painkiller. I had to check painkillers and then suddenly somebody start vomiting so I had to go, you know, and help this patient. So I am supposed to say I am going to toilet, I will be back in five minutes? You can't explain I need to go to toilet, I'll help you in five minutes. She was sick.

The pace of the ward can often feel uncomfortable, operating a fine line between safe and dangerous:

Amelia: It is scary sometimes, because you think you are going to miss something; that you are not going to pick something up, and you know that could be somebody's life. But you also feel that; well, I feel that I have the insight to know that I am not perfect, I am only human and I will forget things and I will not do things and I can't help that. Not when sometimes you have got so many things to do, you can't remember everything.

These challenges often leave the nurses feeling frustrated with how much work they still have to do and aware of the lack of time they give to their patients.

Maxine: I think that this job is mainly feeling guilty isn't it? It's all to do with staffing levels, politics, things that I have no control over. And yes you do, I'd say ninety-nine times out of a hundred you do go home feeling guilty, because you are thinking you've not done the care that you should have done or given to that particular group of patients. Instead of achieving the gold standard, you are achieving the bronze standard, which is better than achieving no standard at all I think (*laughter*)!

The challenges can also be motivating and exciting and the work immensely satisfying.

Kay [E grade staff nurse]: Today started badly. We were understaffed by one trained nurse and during handover it emerged that I had an extremely poorly patient. Myself and two HCAs were looking after C, D and E [nineteen patients], and the patient in C6 had become poorly overnight almost requiring one to one nursing. Handover itself took longer than it should do, about forty minutes. Once on the ward I checked the patient and took several observations before starting the drug round. The patient had had an oesophageal gastrectomy four days ago and overnight had dropped his BP [blood pressure] and urine output, and was becoming dyspnoeic despite oxygen therapy. He had stabilised but his BP was still low.

I started the drug round and asked my HCA to concentrate on getting the beds made after breakfast. I was interrupted during the drug round by the doctors attending C6. I spent the next half an hour carrying out their orders. After the drug round I contacted the outreach team as I felt that he needed more input than I could give without neglecting my other patients. Luckily there were no other really poorly patients or too many high dependency ones and I was able to concentrate most of my efforts on C6. While he was off the ward having an investigation, I took my break which I desperately needed at that time. I was able to handover D and E bay to the RGN [registered general nurse] on the afternoon shift and he managed to do any dressings that needed to be done. By 7pm the doctors decided that the patient should be nursed on ITU [Intensive Care Unit] and transferred him. I used the next hour to catch up on paperwork. At 8pm we had an admission from A & E [Accident and Emergency], another poorly patient with suspected perforation, although no one would say of what! She needed a lot of attention on admission as A & E had sent her up to the ward needing catheterisation, IV fluids, NG tube, ECG, IVAB [intravenous fluids, naso-gastric tube, echo-cardio-gram, intravenous antibiotics], etc. I set up IV fluids and catheterised her and while I handed over, the other RGN did the rest. We went off the ward at 9.45pm. Despite things being extremely busy, I enjoyed the day. At times it was frustrating especially trying to get the doctors to make a decision on transfer to ITU. I had a good team of HCAs on the early shift so I was able to leave them to get on with the rest of the ward knowing they would inform me of any problems. It was unsatisfactory in that I didn't have much contact with the rest of my patients.

Ward B is one of the busiest wards in the hospital. Surgery takes place every day. Patients come in for major surgery such as abdominal aortic aneurysm repair (a massive life-saving operation, requiring high dependency nursing); bypass grafts and limb amputations for patients with vascular disease; and minor surgery, such as thyroidectomies, hernia repairs or appendectomies. Although the ward has thirty-four beds, there are usually at least ten discharges and admissions each day, thus, the number of patients cared for daily can be as many as forty-four. However, the number of qualified staff on duty each shift is usually only three. Managing a huge work demand with too few human resources is an everyday problem. The prioritisation of work and the ward routine is essential to maintaining patient safety and wellbeing in the accomplishment of this. Consequently, nurses often have less time to spend with their patients. This can impact on how patients and their relatives experience the care given at a time when they are most vulnerable, and it can seem as if the nurses no longer have a passion for the personal and relational skills of healing (R. Williams 2006).

Wards are emotional places irrespective of the type of care they offer. People are admitted to them because they require some form of care that they are unable to receive at home. That care, which may involve intimate knowledge of their mind, body and everyday lives, takes place in an alien environment with people who are often strangers to them. Emotionally, these people can be extremely vulnerable. So too are their friends and relatives, stripped of their familiar roles and dependent on the knowledge and information that health care professionals pass their way. Both patient and relative are subject to the control of others. The capacity of the health care professional to understand and respect this emotional vulnerability is immensely important. There is, however, a worrying body of literature that suggests that health care professionals, and most especially nurses, are increasingly insensitive to their patients' emotional welfare. Thus, in an address at the annual commemoration of Florence Nightingale, Archbishop Williams (2006) emphasised the need for the profession to retain its commitment to human dignity.

Many reasons for the decrease in nurses' emotional labour have been put forward. Some suggest that emotional labour in nursing has become marginalised due to organisational changes which have resulted in a massive increase in the pace and quantity of nursing work. Nurses are now so busy they have little time for their patients' emotional welfare. Others suggest that emotional labour lacks the status of medical care and so nurses are prioritising the latter because it is considered more important. Again, this results in emotional labour becoming marginalised. Others argue that health care in the UK has become increasingly commercialised, seen as a commodity patients have a right to. This has resulted in nurses becoming increasingly alienated from their own sense of self as emotional labour is demanded from them irrespective of patient needs. Thus, they present a smiling face while suppressing their real feelings of frustration and anger at the degree of abuse hurled at them.

Implicit in all these accounts is a picture of a profession that no longer prioritises the emotional welfare of patients and their relatives. The evidence for this accusation is sufficient to suggest that the nursing profession needs to address it. The implication that nurses have a lack of compassion and respect towards their patients burdens the nurses with more guilt. However, since the emotional needs of patients are real, and since nurses seem to be feeling frustrated, angry and guilty towards them, the question needs to be asked what happens to all these emotions if emotional labour is so absent from nursing care? It seems that there are two answers to this question. The first is that these emotions are not being managed because emotional labour is marginalised, creating increasingly stressful environments for patients and nurses alike. The reasons for this, the nursing profession has a responsibility to address. The second is that the emotional labour carried out is largely invisible, either because it is misunderstood or because the nature of emotional labour in nursing care has changed and developed alongside nursing work, becoming unrecognisable. Either way it seems that it is necessary to re-examine and understand the nature of emotional labour in nursing today in order to understand how the profession can redress current concerns and/or to identify how emotional labour might have changed and developed. This is the aim of the research presented in this book.

The challenge has been how to go about achieving it without reproducing the work and findings of others. The answer to this forms two main objectives underpinning the purpose of this research. The first is concerned with developing understanding of the *concept* of emotional labour by examining its relationship with emotion. The second is to apply that concept to nursing and analyse the implications of the findings that result from it. To do this, in Part I of the book, theoretical approaches towards emotion and emotional labour are analysed and reflected through the lens of empirical data collected specifically for this purpose. In Part II, that process is reversed, and the empirical data are analysed and reflected through the lens of the theoretical approaches discussed in Part I. Two major themes run throughout, connecting Parts I and II. The first is that the purpose of emotional labour is the management of emotion. *Emotion* is the driving force and focus behind this study. In Part I, an attempt is made to theoretically understand its nature in as full a manner as possible, in order to better understand the character of emotional labour. In Part II, an attempt is made to identify emotion and retain 'the emotional' in the analysis of the empirical data. The second theme is that emotional labour takes place in context. The context in this case is Ward B where the empirical data collection took place. Accessing and uncovering the emotion experiences and the emotional labour carried out by the nurses in order to understand them is pivotal to all aspects of this book. The aim of the empirical data collection, therefore, was to experience and capture the emotions and emotional labour carried out by the qualified nursing staff as they naturally occurred within the nursing context. The data are represented throughout the book in vignettes preceding each chapter. In Part I, although the focus is theoretical, the reality of the lived experience of the nurses' emotion and emotional labour represented in the vignettes is reflected and applied to the theoretical discourse. In Part II, those experiences are the focus of the analysis, and inform the conclusions drawn from them. The research presented in this book, therefore, is a theoretically informed empirical analysis of the relationship between emotion and emotional labour as experienced by nurses on an acute vascular surgical ward. In taking this approach, it is hoped that the book will be useful to sociologists, interested in the study of emotion, and nurses interested in the application of emotional labour to nursing.

The empirical data collection took place over a period of fourteen months from August 2000 to October 2001 when I worked on Ward B as a D grade staff nurse. Ethical consent was gained from the Local Research Ethics Committee, the nursing research committee, the Nursing Director of the NHS Trust and the G grade sister on Ward B. From the beginning, all members of staff knew I was there to carry out research in addition to my nursing duties. There was a high turnover of staff in that period, but fifteen qualified nurses (fourteen female and one male) consented to record audio diaries and be interviewed about their experiences, feelings and opinions of life on Ward B. The nurses have all been given pseudonyms in order to protect their identity. I also recorded my own personal audio diary which documented my observations and experiences as a staff nurse there. The accounts represented in the vignettes are drawn from the diaries, interviews and participant observation. A table of the vignettes identifying who the nurses are, and the source of their narrative, can be found on page xi.

The emotional stories encapsulated in the vignettes are often unwieldy and may feel shocking. The nurses graphically illustrated their emotions and feelings in order to describe the situations they found themselves in; thus, their feelings emerge and are dramatised as they weave their stories explaining what has happened to them. The accounts in the vignettes are therefore largely unedited except where it is absolutely necessary for understanding. Their narratives may also seem shocking because they represent a side of nursing rarely shared outside the profession. There is little evidence of the professional face of nursing here. This does not mean that the care carried out on Ward B was poor. Rather it represents their particular perceptions of nursing and their relationships with their patients, relatives and colleagues during this period of time, which were shared with someone who worked with them. I am wholly indebted to the nurses for agreeing to participate and for doing so with frankness, honesty and integrity. A full account of the methodology and the context can be found in Chapter 6 at the beginning of Part II.

Throughout the book you are invited to engage with the nurses, in an emotional and theoretical exploration of their emotions and emotional labour. Part I begins by introducing the concept of emotional labour.

Part I

Understanding emotional labour in nursing

A theoretical approach

Vignette 1 'Half measures'

Catherine: What would you describe as good care that gives you satisfaction?

Paris: Good care: obviously clinically I would be able to look after my patients properly. But, psychologically, I could spend time with them and see what their fears are, what their worries are; to give them good pain control so that they are not in pain. I don't think we do it half the time. We are running the ward, and it is one of the most stressful wards as far as the patients are concerned because the majority of them, they come for major surgery. They come for aneurysm repair, bypass, they come for cancer. How many times do we get to tell them about their operation? How many times? We count it on our hand. I don't do it enough. I admit you I don't, because I am too conscious about not letting the next lady dehydrate and not leaving the other man in pain. You constantly want to see that everybody's need has been met halfway. Because I feel if I could go and give proper pre-op care, and sit with the patient for half an hour and the wife and the son and the daughter and answer their questions and make sure that psychologically they are cared for, then I have neglected somebody else's pain or somebody else's dressing or somebody has dehydrated because the fluid has been behind for six hours. What I do, which I am not happy about, is I try and meet everybody's needs halfway. So I know that he is moderately hydrated and that the IV is not behind three or four hours. I know that this patient has had all his oral analgesia, the dressing has been done, so he is not in pain because of his wound. But that is not good enough because the psychological care has gone out of the window. When I was a third year student – because I had more time, because I didn't have responsibilities and accountabilities – I had time to spend with the patient. Every cancer patient, Catherine, the doctor who went and told them about their diagnosis and prognosis, I remember, every single one of them. I pulled the curtain around and I sat with them, and I said, 'Did you understand what he said?' I asked what their worries were. I went through with them what was going to happen, what was their after care. What their referrals were. They would say, 'Who is Dr Smitt?' you know, and I would tell them. And then I would leave them and then go back twenty minutes, half an hour later to see how they were coping, if they had any more questions to ask. I'd call the Macmillan nurse, call this and call that. I haven't done that since I qualified. I don't remember, maybe as a D grade I did a few, but not since I made E grade. So many times I have just burst into tears because of this situation and we do get involved a lot, especially if they are young. I have done this, six or seven times in handover, because the lady was dying. But it didn't help her. I think: 'So what? I got emotional but did it help her? Did I sit and talk to her about how she feels?' No, I didn't. As long as the patients are washed and they are in clean beds, that is all that matters now. They can be having the most difficult time of their life, thinking about what the doctors have told them without any nurses going to see how they feel, if they have any questions. That is not nursing care, it is total crap.

1 Emotion management and emotional labour

The work of Arlie Russell Hochschild

The term emotional labour was first coined by the American sociologist Arlie Russell Hochschild (1975, 1979, 1983, 1990). She carried out extensive research in the airline industry, particularly focusing on the emotion work of flight attendants. Hochschild's work is considered to be groundbreaking in understanding the significance of emotion to everyday life for individuals, families and in the workplace. Most research examining emotional labour draws on her original ideas and concepts. To understand how emotional labour in nursing and health care has developed, it is necessary to explore Hochschild's work first and then consider how it relates to health care. The aim of this chapter therefore is to introduce and explore Hochschild's work; unpacking and discussing what she means by emotion management, feeling rules, surface acting, deep acting and emotional labour. The chapter is written so the relationship between Hochschild's ideas can be clearly followed as they develop. As the concepts are introduced, their relevance to nursing is directly applied to Vignette 1 'Half measures'. This narrative is taken from my interview with Paris, an F grade junior sister on Ward B. The applications of Hochschild's ideas are considered at the end of each section: their relevance is identified without interrupting the account of her work. Thus, this chapter explores Hochschild's work and considers whether her key ideas are reflected within nursing experience.

Hochschild's background

As a child, Hochschild was fascinated by the work of her parents, who were US Foreign Service diplomats. Her interest in emotion management began as a child when she was invited to pass drinks and nibbles around the visiting foreign dignitaries. Every gesture and smile was closely monitored and interpreted for hidden meanings. She writes:

> Afterwards I would listen to my mother and father interpret various gestures. The tight smile of the Bulgarian emissary, the averted glance of the Chinese consul, the prolonged handshake of the French economic officer, I learned, conveyed messages not simply from person to person

but from Sofia to Washington, from Peking to Paris and from Paris to Washington. Had I passed the peanuts to a person, I wondered, or an actor? Where did the person end and the act begin? Just how is a person related to an act?

(Hochschild 1983: ix)

This fascination led Hochschild to explore the relationship between emotions that are really felt and the ones that are acted out for the benefit of others. For her, this is an inherently social act, because in order to work out what emotions individuals should perform, they need to be able to understand the social context in which they are actors. For example, it is socially acceptable to cry at a funeral and laugh at a party even if the person feels hysterical at the funeral and sad at the party. Thus, the social context, funeral or party, dictates what emotion they should act out even if this is different from what they really feel.

Later, as a graduate student at Berkeley, University of California, Hochschild read C. Wright Mills' influential book *White Collar* (1951). He argued that in the world of sales, the sales process is as much about the personality of the sales person as it is about the product being sold. In fact, Mills argued that in the sales process the sales people were actually selling their personality. Mills felt that this could be detrimental to the sales people because it resulted in them becoming estranged from themselves. These ideas appealed to Hochschild. However, she felt that there was something missing in his account. In the preface to her book *The Managed Heart*, she notes:

Mills seemed to assume that in order to sell personality one need only have it. Yet simply having a personality does not make one a diplomat, any more than having muscles makes one an athlete. What was missing was a sense of the active emotional labour involved in selling.

(Hochschild 1983: ix)

Hochschild directly identifies the importance of knowing how to use one's personality, or more specifically, one's emotions in the selling process. In essence, Hochschild's work brings together these ideas about emotion management, acting, the social context and selling one's personal emotions in the labour market as if they were a product.

Emotion management

Hochschild (1983: 7) defines emotion management as 'the management of feeling to create a publicly observable facial and bodily display'. Children learn how to do this through socialisation processes as they grow up. For example, pictures often show young children learning how to express surprise or being taught to control their tears when they are unhappy.

Emotion management requires emotion *work*, because learning how to do it takes effort. For example, when little Johnny feels disappointment at receiving a hand-knitted cardigan from his grandmother instead of the shiny red toy truck he was hoping for, his mother teaches him to show pleasure and gratitude instead of tears and a tantrum. She may have to take him aside, allowing him time to control his feelings, then explain that he should go up to his grandmother, give her a kiss and say thank you for his lovely cardigan. In this way, Johnny learns not only how to control his emotions, but also what emotions he ought to be expressing in this situation (feeling rules). Thus, he learns that he should manage his disappointment and instead display pleasure and gratitude which he enacts for the benefit of his grandmother and his mother.

In learning this, Johnny also realises that there is a difference between his real private feelings and what he can express publicly. The difference between the *private* and *public* sphere is fundamental to Hochschild's differing notions of emotion management and emotional labour. Here she draws on the work of Erving Goffman (1956, 1959, 1961, 1967, 1969, 1974), who examined how people know how to behave and how they present themselves to others in everyday public life. He drew on the analogy of the theatre in order to help explain everyday interaction. One of the important distinctions Goffman (1959) made is the difference between *front stage* and *back stage*. The front stage is where performance takes place, where a show is put on. An example given here is the role of the waitress being pleasant and polite to the customers, enquiring what they want to eat and if she can help them in anyway. When she returns to the kitchen, in the back stage, she might bad mouth them to her colleagues working behind the scenes. Hochschild uses this distinction in her work, seeing emotion work as belonging in the private realm (at home or back stage) and emotional labour as belonging in the public realm (in the workplace or front stage). This private/public distinction, however, is not as clear cut as Hochschild presents it (Wouters 1989a, 1989b, 1991). For her, where and why emotion management occurs creates the fundamental difference between the two. In the private realm, emotion work is considered as being a part of our private lives and takes place in the home; whereas emotional labour is sold for a wage as a commodity and takes place at work. It is an important distinction for Hochschild because it represents the exploitation to which she feels emotional labourers are subjected. However, as is seen in the illustration of Johnny and his mother and grandmother, front and back stage life can coexist together in the private realm, and as seen in the example of waitress, in the public one. In many ways, the distinction is really one of a difference of self, between what individuals consider belongs to them, representing their 'real selves', and what is socially acceptable and for public consumption. Hochschild's notion of feeling rules is much more helpful in this respect.

Emotion management in 'Half measures' (Vignette 1)

The basic principle of emotion management can be identified in Paris' vignette 'Half measures'. Paris tells us what it is that she is really feeling in respect to her dying lady. She is upset and this causes her to cry. When she is with her patient (front stage), she manages her feelings and displays a more appropriate face. This is emotion management. However, she tells us that she did cry in handover (back stage). On the ward there are areas that are accessible only to the nursing staff. This represents their 'back stage' areas. Handover on Ward B took place in the nurses' staff room. It is here that Paris feels free to display her real emotions.

Paris implies that emotion management and front and back stage also applies to her patients. When she explains good nursing care, she describes how she would draw the curtains around the patient and their relatives in order to create a private place (back stage) for them in which they can express their real feelings to her. An implication here could be that when they are on the front stage, with the curtains open, they are less likely to express their real feelings; rather they manage them and express emotions that are more appropriate in a public place.

Feeling rules

Feeling rules represent *what* emotions people should express and *the degree* of that expression according to their social roles:

> Acts of emotion management are not simply private acts; they are used in exchanges under the guidance of feeling rules. Feeling rules are standards used in emotional conversation to determine what is rightly owed in the currency of feeling. Through them, we tell what is 'due' in each relation, each role. We pay tribute to each other in the currency of the managing act. In interaction we pay, overpay, underpay, play with paying, acknowledge our due, pretend to pay, or acknowledge what is emotionally due another person.
>
> (Hochschild 1983: 18)

This can be seen in the example of little Johnny earlier. His grandmother expended emotional energy, as well as time and money, in making the cardigan for him. When she takes him aside, his mother explains that he is required to express gratitude for, and pleasure in, the gift his grandmother has given him. This is the feeling rule: on receipt of a gift it is right to express thanks and pleasure irrespective of whether those feelings are real. Individuals learn to hide disappointment and show excitement and love, and ultimately, to return the favour in giving them a gift too. Individuals learn how to show these emotions in respect to their relationship with the other person. When it is a lover, they might express their thanks differently from when it is a friend, colleague, neighbour or parent. Johnny's relationship with his grandmother is special, and in his role as grandson he is expected to show her deference and love.

Feeling rules also help identify and define what the emotions being experienced are. When Johnny burst into tears on unwrapping a cardigan instead of the hoped-for toy truck, the emotion he experienced can be interpreted as disappointment because his anticipated pleasure in getting a toy truck was thwarted. Rather than his feelings just being a bodily sensation, therefore, they have meaning according to the social circumstances in which they occur. Feeling rules are the means through which individuals understand what the emotions they feel are, and they are the means by which they know what emotions they should express and to what degree they should express them.

Feeling rules in 'Half measures' (Vignette 1)

The question posed at the beginning of Vignette 1 'What would you describe as good care that gives you satisfaction?' suggests that good care elicits an emotional response of satisfaction. This is indicative of a feeling rule: the giving of good care produces feelings of satisfaction in the carer. Paris identifies this feeling rule immediately: 'obviously clinically I would be able to look after my patients properly. But, psychologically . . .'. Paris suggests that in nursing, the feeling rule about giving good care includes both the physical and psychological care: it is this that is satisfying to the nurse. Paris implies that she 'owes' her patients psychological care, and she expresses dissatisfaction when she cannot carry this out, suggesting that the care she gives can only 'meet everybody's needs halfway'. In fact Paris is so dissatisfied with the care she gives, that she states that it is not even 'nursing care' at all, rather it is 'total crap'. That good nursing care involves both the physical and the psychological, is an ideal, by which she measures and judges her own nursing performance.

Paris also points out another feeling rule when she says that patients 'can be having the most difficult time of their life, thinking about what the doctors have told them without any nurses going to see how they feel, if they have any questions'. This is a feeling rule from the patient's point of view. The doctors tell them about their medical condition but the nurses interpret what that means and deal with feelings that result from it. This feeling rule suggests that patients can expect this kind of care from the nurses, and Paris suggests that this is what she feels she owes them.

Paris identifies a further feeling rule: that it is not helpful for the patient if the nurse becomes too involved and expresses her feelings about her patient's situation. It is the nurse's role to suppress her feelings on behalf of her patient in order to help them. Paris implies, however, that nurses get involved anyway.

Surface and deep acting

How then do people manage their emotions? Drawing on the work of method actor Constantin Stanislavski, and extending Goffman's metaphor of the theatre, Hochschild suggests that individuals manage their emotions through surface and deep acting. She defines surface acting as 'the ability to deceive others about how we are really feeling without deceiving ourselves'. This is in contrast to deep acting where 'we deceive ourselves about our true emotion as much as we deceive others' (Hochschild 1983: 33). In surface acting, the individual uses their body to portray feelings that they do not really have, by smiling, shrugging, sneering and laughing. The actor knows they are pretending. For example, when an individual is with a group of friends and a joke is told, they might make a great show of laughing and finding the joke very funny even if the opposite is true. They use their face and whole body to portray amusement and laugh in order to enter into the group spirit of fun and enjoyment.

In deep acting, however, Hochschild suggests that the actor learns to really believe in the emotions they are expressing through 'conscious mental work'. 'Here display is a natural result of working on feeling; the actor does not try to seem happy or sad but rather expresses spontaneously . . . a real feeling that has been self induced' (Hochschild 1983: 35). There are two ways in which an actor can do deep acting. One is by exhorting emotion and the other is by using their imagination. People exhort feelings all the time. For example, a person might 'psyche' themselves up to do something they are not looking forward to, or 'get into the party frame of mind' looking to enjoy themselves when they go out. This is part of what Johnny is being taught by his mother. It is possible to imagine him controlling his tears, while his mother points out:

> What a lovely cardigan Johnny! Grandma knitted that especially for you. I bet there are no other boys with such a lovely cardigan with a bright red digger on it. You will be able to show it off to all your friends!

This stream of advice demonstrates a practical way of exhorting 'proper' emotions of pleasure and gratitude.

Hochschild also notes that deep acting can be the result of training one's imagination. Here individuals draw on their emotion memory, imagining how they could act out more appropriate emotions. For example, Johnny's mother could say to him:

> Do you remember how excited you were when you made that lovely picture for me of our house, and how much work you put into it so that it would be special? Can you remember how you felt when I was so pleased you made it especially for me? I expect Grandma felt just like you did when she was making that cardigan for you.

Here, through use of both emotion memory and imagination, Johnny is encouraged to remember his feelings of pleasure and excitement when he gave his mother a gift, and to transfer those feelings to the current situation using his imagination. Through such deep acting, Johnny's feelings can be worked on to produce the proper responses. Hochschild believes that eventually a person can learn to do this so well, that they *really* believe the feelings that deep acting produces, unaware that they have *worked* on them and *created* the required feeling expression.

Private emotion management, therefore, is something that becomes associated with the individual's sense of self, their emotion memories and imagination. It is acted out according to the currency of feeling they believe they owe their friends and family – and through this can be linked with their sense of identity. But, Hochschild asks, what happens then when their private emotions and their emotion work is used in the workplace?

Surface and deep acting in 'Half measures' (Vignette 1)

Surface and deep acting is much harder to see directly in Vignette 1; there are however, some glimpses of both, implicit in the examples Paris uses to explain what she feels is good, satisfying nursing care.

Surface acting is implicit within Paris' suggestion that nursing care that attempts to meet all patients' needs 'halfway' is neither good quality care nor satisfying to the nurse. In fact, Paris notes that in the case of terminal patients, these 'halfway' measures are enough to bring her to tears. But, she says, 'So what? I got emotional but did it help her?' This implies that in the care that Paris gives, she is surface acting, presenting a 'professional face' to the patients and their relatives, while privately acknowledging her own discomfort and distress over the care being given.

Deep acting is evident in Paris' example of what good care that results in satisfaction for the nurse, is. She explains that when she was a third year student and junior staff nurse she had more time to give to her patients. Consequently, she was able to spend time listening to them, encouraging them to express their feelings. In her explanation of this, she illustrates and draws on her emotion memory which elicits the feeling of satisfaction associated with good care. She gives details about closing the curtains around them, she even remembers the name of the consultant, she recalls that she referred them to the Macmillan nurse and that she went back to them twenty or thirty minutes later to check how they were doing and if they had any further questions or anxieties. This is suggestive of deep acting. However, it has also become a template by which she measures the degree of her feelings when she cannot give this kind of care. This emotion memory has become so embedded that it can cause her to cry with distress.

Emotional labour

The basis of Hochschild's argument is that in the workplace private emotion management or work is exploited for commercial purposes. Using interviews and observation, Hochschild explored the emotional labour of flight attendants and bill collectors working with Delta Airlines. She found that flight attendants are carefully recruited and trained to sell the flight company through a carefully prescribed image. The image that Delta Airlines portrayed was one of Southern charm and hospitality, used to encourage the passengers to feel relaxed, safe and comfortable on their journey. This image was portrayed by the flight attendants through their physical image and through the emotion work they carried out.

The process of learning emotional labour started with recruitment. Here the company set out to identify people who can 'project a warm personality' and who can 'convey a spirit of enthusiasm' (Hochschild 1983: 97). During intensive training, the flight attendants were taught to receive the passengers on to the plane as if they were guests in their own home – in effect to act out the idea of Southern charm and hospitality. They were expected always to smile, to make the passengers feel safe and comfortable – to act as a hostess. Learning that the passenger is always right, and that the flight attendant must always control her emotions for their benefit by producing a happy smiling face, is a central part of the feeling rules introduced, taught and monitored during training. In this way, the flight attendants' private emotion work undergoes what Hochschild calls transmutation, becoming emotional labour. Emotional labour, therefore, is emotion work used in the workplace for commercial value. It is:

> Labour that requires one to induce or suppress feeling in order to sustain the outward countenance that produces the proper state of mind in others [such as] the sense of being cared for in a convivial and safe place. This kind of labour calls for a coordination of mind and feeling, and it sometimes draws on a source of self that we honour as deep and

integral to our individuality . . . Emotional labour is sold for a wage and therefore has exchange value.

(Hochschild 1983: 7)

The purpose of emotional labour is to promote a good company image, which persuades customers to believe that they receive a warm and friendly service from Delta Airlines, thereby encouraging them to use the company's services. Emotional labour therefore results in 'bums on seats' and greater profit for the airline company.

Emotional labour in 'Half measures' (Vignette 1)

The emotion management that Paris describes in Vignette 1 takes place at work in her role as an F grade junior sister, for which she receives a wage: it is emotional labour. An essential part of emotional labour in nursing is to encourage patients to feel safe and to trust the care that is being given to them.

There are many other aspects of Hochschild's notion of emotional labour in this vignette, but many of them are hidden, taken-for-granted parts. For example, the feeling rule identified earlier expresses the ideal that nurses care for the psychological needs of the patients as well as their physical ones. Such nursing care includes the emotional needs of the patient, and it is this that is considered to be satisfying. This feeling rule is linked to an 'ideal' image of the nurse as intrinsically kind and caring, choosing to nurse others because it is something that she considers worthwhile and personally satisfying.

That Paris can carry out both surface and, particularly, deep acting suggests that she has been carefully taught how to do so. When she describes the actions she would take when giving emotional care, she mentions many factors indicative of a nurse's interpersonal and communication skills – a subject taught and monitored during nurse training. In fact, she also notes that as a student she was more likely to carry this out. She identifies the importance of drawing the curtains round the patient, demonstrating an awareness of their need for privacy. It also shows that she is giving them a space in which to explore and express their feelings. She encourages them to talk to her, and shows her willingness to give her time and energy to listening and understanding. But most importantly she puts herself in their shoes, saying 'it is one of the most stressful wards as far as the patients are concerned' and 'They can be having the most difficult time of their life'. In college, encouraging the student to imagine what their patient might be feeling as a result of their illness and hospital admission is strongly encouraged. This helps them to feel empathy for their patients.

Inauthenticity of self

Hochschild sets her concept of emotional labour in the capitalist discourse where it has commodity value and is controlled by the company who the labourer works for. The motivation for emotional labour is one of profit. However, the process of carrying out emotional labour draws on an individual's sense of self. She argues that this creates a division between the 'real/true self' and the 'false self' which has consequences for what the individual (and society as a whole) perceives as being authentic emotion. She writes:

> A nineteenth century child working in a brutalising English wallpaper factory and a well paid twentieth century American flight attendant have something in common: in order to do their jobs they must mentally detach themselves – the factory worker from his own body and physical labour and the flight attendant from her own feelings and emotional labour.
>
> (Hochschild 1983: 17)

Private emotion management and deep acting draw on a sense of self that is integral to a person's individuality because it is linked to their emotion memories, imagination and private relationships. However, emotional labour draws on that individuality for commercial purposes, thus individuals are taught feeling rules prescribed and monitored by the company, which encourage them to suppress or deny their real feelings, resulting in them being alienated from their sense of self.

Organisations that require emotional labour, therefore, subvert the worker's 'true self' by reinterpreting the emotions they naturally feel in work situations. For example, in flight attendants' training classes, the students are told that when they feel angry with a difficult passenger, it is because they are wrongly focusing on themselves. Instead, they are encouraged to look at the situation from the passenger's point of view. This effectively means that not only do flight attendants have to deny their own feelings, but also their feelings are not even considered to be justifiable. Consequently, it is their responsibility to work hard at controlling them. As a result, 'the worker may lose touch with her feelings as in burnout, or she may have to struggle with the company interpretation of what they mean' (Hochschild 1983: 197). The cost of emotional labour therefore is one of alienation. This cost was exacerbated when the airline industry went through a 'speed-up'.

Speed-up in the airline industry occurred when there was mass expansion. This expansion meant longer flights, larger aircrafts and many, many more passengers, often flying on budget tickets. Consequently, the flight attendants found that they had little time to be engaging with their passengers and carrying out emotional labour. Because the company's motivation was profit, when this was achieved through different means, the importance of

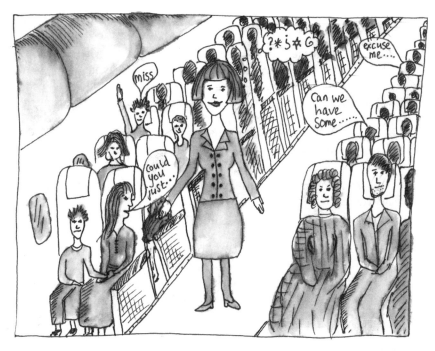

'Speed-up!'

emotional labour also decreased. The flight attendants, however, were still expected to carry out effective emotional labour as part of the service offered. Hochschild felt that this impacted on the flight attendants' sense of self in three different ways.

First, Hochschild found that because their deep acting was so successful, some flight attendants overidentified with their work, seeing their own identity as inextricable from the image that the company set out to portray. This resulted in their being unable to distinguish clearly between themselves and the job, becoming more vulnerable to burnout and stress when speed-up occurred. Second, some flight attendants successfully separated themselves from the role as a flight attendant, but blamed themselves for being able only to surface act, making them feel deficient and insincere, and consequently alienated from their work. Third, Hochschild found that in addition to distinguishing themselves from the act of emotional labour, some flight attendants also became estranged from the acting itself, seeing themselves as illusion makers: they became cynical and alienated from their sense of self as well as from their work. This led Hochschild to the conclusion that the commodification of emotional labour for profit ultimately alienates the worker, resulting in inauthentic emotion expression and a loss of the individual's 'real' sense of self.

Inauthenticity of self in 'Half measures' (Vignette 1)

Nursing has become much busier and faster paced. The patient's physical needs are often very immediate, thus Paris feels she is making do trying to meet all their physical needs at least halfway. The emotional needs of the patients are the ones that are increasingly compromised. They are less tangible and therefore less measurable, whereas the physical needs are immediate and much more obvious. Thus, Paris says with great feeling:

> We are running the ward, and it is one of the most stressful wards as far as the patients are concerned because the majority of them, they come for major surgery. They come for aneurysm repair, bypass, they come for cancer. How many times do we get to tell them about their operation? How many times? We count it on our hand. I don't do it enough. I admit you I don't, because I am too conscious about not letting the next lady dehydrate and not leaving the other man in pain. You constantly want to see that everybody's need has been met halfway.

The underlying message at the heart of Paris' account is one of dissatisfaction, caused by a lack of time to carry out good quality nursing care. This was so distressing that it brought an experienced sister to tears, provoking her into calling her nursing care 'total crap'. This reduction in emotional labour has resulted in an inauthenticity of emotion expression and, consequently, dissatisfaction at work.

Emotional labour and gender

For Hochschild, emotion work and emotional labour are expressly tied to women's work and are illustrative of wider social structures that reflect social status and power. Hochschild believes that women undertake more emotion work in the home than men because they offer it to the men like a gift. This is because they are dependent on them for their material support. Women, therefore, do extra emotion work to offset their financial debt to men. She also suggests that it is women who predominantly nurture, care and manage children. Women's use of emotion work in both these roles is supported by social values and beliefs that women are naturally more emotional than men, and are more likely to be emotionally giving, nurturing and caring. Men, on the other hand, are considered to be more rational, single-minded and level-headed. When they do express emotions they are likely to be more masculine emotions such as aggression and anger.

Hochschild notes that these values are translated into the workplace. In their emotional labour, women are asked to be motherly, supportive and affirming to men. In the workplace, women's subordination to men is also more apparent: it is clearly seen in the different feeling status in the emotional labour they carry out. For example, female flight attendants are accorded little authority and are often subject to verbal and/or physical aggression by passengers. In such situations, a male colleague would be brought in to deal with the situation because the passenger would behave more deferentially towards him. This is due to the authority that men are deemed to have over women, and to the different status accorded to men and women's emotions.

> When a man expresses anger, it is deemed 'rational' or understandable anger, anger that indicates not weakness of character but deeply held conviction. When a woman expresses anger, it is more likely to be interpreted as a sign of personal instability. It is believed that women are more emotional, and this very belief is used to invalidate their feelings. That is, the women's feelings are not seen as a response to real events, but as a reflection of themselves as 'emotional' women.
>
> (Hochschild 1983: 173)

Consequently, Hochschild found that the female flight attendants were infinitely more exposed to rudeness, bigotry and rough treatment than their male counterparts.

While women's emotional relational abilities are primarily exploited for commercial purposes in emotional labour, Hochschild suggests that their emotional labour was accorded little status and respect. Thus, when the airline industry went through speed-up, emotional labour was given a very low priority, making the female flight attendants even more vulnerable to a loss of self, inauthenticity in their emotional labour and a sense of dismissal concerning their own feelings.

Emotional labour and gender in 'Half measures'
(Vignette 1)

Nurses are predominantly female. On Ward B there was only one male nurse, reflecting this. As a consequence, it is not possible to carry out gender analysis in this book. However, Hochschild is talking about more than the situational effect of gender. She also links emotional labour to social status and describes emotion as being given gendered characteristics. There are several indications of this in Paris' vignette.

Underpinning the complaint that there is no time to carry out emotional labour is the assumption that the physical and clinical side of nursing is more important. At heart, it could be suggested that the clinical side of nursing, linked to the scientific approach of medicine, which is rational and more masculine, is prioritised because it has a higher status value. This is also reflected in the status difference between the medical and nursing professions. Because greater status is given to the biomedical, there is a corresponding assumption that the patient's physical needs always outweigh emotional and psychological ones. This is emphasised in the fact that the nurse's clinical role has been largely developed and extended from previous medical responsibilities. As a nurse travels up the career scale, her role becomes more clinically specialised (in addition to her managerial responsibilities). Thus, Paris notes that when she was a student nurse and even as a junior staff nurse, she had more time to give to emotional labour. Now, when a conflict occurs between the patient's physical and psychological needs, Paris genuinely believes the physical ones have a greater priority. This results in her neglecting the patient's emotional care, creating dissatisfaction in Paris, and a deficit of care need in the patient.

The significance of emotional labour

Hochschild's work has enormous value, not least because her account of private emotion management, its commercial exploitation and its impact on women in the workplace is very compelling. More significant however, is that Hochschild's account of emotion management in its very conceptualisation and identification demonstrates an inherently social manifestation of emotion. Not only does she successfully identify and define the significance of emotion to understanding social life, but also she shows how emotion can be shaped, even created (through inducing and exhorting) for social purposes. In her concept of feeling rules, she also makes emotion empirically more observable, identifiable and definable, and it is this in combination with clearly defined concepts of the social nature of emotion which has been so essential in furthering the sociology of emotion.

Unsurprisingly, her ideas have been taken up by many others trying to understand the significance of emotion, emotion management and emotional labour to social life. This chapter has also introduced how Hochschild's work is relevant to nursing today by reflecting her ideas and concepts through Paris' narrative. In Chapter 2 the relevance of emotional labour to nursing is investigated in more detail, exploring how other writers in the field of health care have taken up, applied and interpreted Hochschild's notion of emotional labour.

Vignette 2 'Alix's dad'

Amelia *(from audio diary)*: Alix's dad is causing a few problems. I think, I don't know if it's his manner or if it's just the way he speaks to you. Yesterday I said to him: 'I've put a pad on Alix, because I'm sure he is going to have his bowels open because when we were changing him he seemed to be'. So we had just finished handing over in the afternoon, and the father came out and he said: 'You had better get in there and change him because he's putting his hands in it!' [imperiously] Well we didn't even know that he'd been incontinent yet! So I mean if he had just let us know and come out and said, 'Excuse me, do you mind coming in and changing him' [said politely], we would have done it right away. It's just people like that just make you so angry when they are so rude.

Catherine (from interview): Can you sort of expand on what happened in this incident with Alix's dad?

Well, the first day that Alix was there, I went in – and I had not seen the parents before – and I went in and we washed him all over. And I said to them: 'He has got that old pyjama jacket on because we couldn't find another T-shirt to put on', really sort of friendly and nice and *he* [the father] turned round to me and said: 'Why hasn't he got pad and pants on?' [demanding angry voice used] And Alix hadn't had pad and pants on when I went in there earlier and I'd not seen him before, so I said: 'Oh that's fine if you want me to put pad and pants on him that's fine'. And that was the attitude, it wasn't, 'Oh don't worry about the pyjama jacket and by the way why hasn't he got pad and pants on?' [friendly conversational tone] It was 'Why hasn't he got pad and pants on?' [demanding] And that was the dad's attitude you know, that sort of confrontational right from the start. And the other day [two months later], you know, Pippa [HCA] and I, 'cos you know what Alix is like when he pees, he just floods the bed. Now Pippa and I had washed him, and we hadn't washed him half an hour and put him clean sheets and everything on him, and they went in there and of course he was soaking again. And it was, 'Why hasn't he been changed?' and Pippa said: 'Well, we have actually just done him', but they wouldn't believe us, they don't believe you. So it's sort of, I just feel that his [the father's] attitude is a little bit, you know. And I mean we don't know when someone is going to have their bowels opened! Nobody actually told us when he had, it was like, 'Why isn't he changed? Why don't you come and change him?' and we didn't even know he was dirty, you know, we're not psychic! They seem to think you're psychic as well don't they? And he was putting his hands in it and they were in there. Why were they letting him put his hands in it?

Does it make you feel defensive?

It does yes. Yes, it does, yes, very. I think, well, I don't like you mate, I don't like you! But you get that attitude a lot, you know. Mum is all right, but Dad is just, I think he has a lot of problems. You try and put yourself in their position, and it *is* terrible what is happening. But there again you find, and I think if they thought about it, you'd get much more response and much more cooperation if you are pleasant to people, you know.

We have lots of head injuries here. And you find that the ones like Ben – I don't know if you remember him, he was a young chap who fell out of a window – and his parents were wonderful and they cooperated with the staff and you find that if they can cooperate they get a lot better. I am saying that they get more and better attention, I'm saying that because if, when you walk into a room and people are aggressive, watching everything you do and criticising everything you do, and writing down everything, then you don't go in there. You just don't go in there and try and build up a rapport with people. But if people are pleasant with you and you go in and you say, 'Well I'm going to do this' and they either go out or stay in or whatever, it doesn't bother me, and they sort of cooperate with you. I think that the patient gets better care because you don't mind going in the room. You don't feel that you are going to go into the room and, well literally I mean you know what some of them are like, they watch every move you make don't they? They even write it down sometimes what you are doing.

2 Emotional labour in health care

Hochschild never applied emotional labour to nursing herself. She does acknowledge, however, that emotional labour as an aspect of paid work can apply to other forms of employment. Such jobs must meet certain criteria:

> First, they require face-to-face or voice-to-voice contact with the public. Second, they require the worker to produce an emotional state in another person – gratitude or fear for example. Third, they allow the employer, through training and supervision to exercise a degree of control over the emotional activities of employees.
>
> (Hochschild 1983: 147)

Drawing on these three characteristics, others have applied her ideas to many areas of work and employment; emotional labour has been found to be particularly relevant to the health and social care professions:

> [M]any professional workers – counsellors, doctors, nurses, social workers and the like – are also, in effect, paid for their emotion management. They are to look serious, understanding, controlled, cool, empathetic and so forth with their clients or patients. The feeling rules are implicit in their professional 'discipline' (an apt term) – 'rational', 'scientific', 'caring', 'objective'. Benign detachment disguises, and defends against, any private feelings of pain, despair, fear, attraction, revulsion or love, feelings which would otherwise interfere with their professional relationship.
>
> (Fineman 1993: 19)

Hochschild's criteria apply to nursing. For example, all nursing work involves face-to-face or voice-to-voice interaction except in cases where patients are unconscious. Even when caring for unconscious patients, it is assumed that they may be aware of the presence of others and able to hear what is being said to them. Nursing work also requires nurses to consider the feelings and emotions of their patients (and their relatives), to engender feelings of safety and comfort, caring and protecting their dignity at all times.

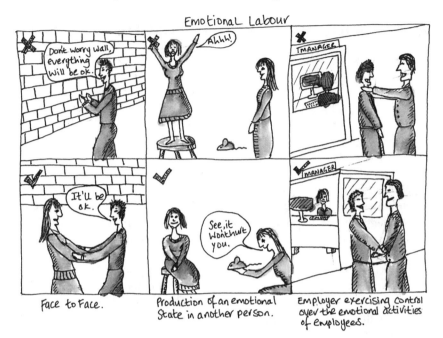

'Characteristics of emotional labour'

Qualified nurses are bound by the Nursing and Midwifery Council (NMC) Code of Conduct, which specifies their role as patient's advocate. The emotional care that nurses give is carefully taught during nurse training and is monitored in a variety of ways. Pam Smith (1992) was one of the first to specifically identify the relevance of emotional labour to nursing and particularly to student nurses. In fact she went to California to study under Hochschild. Smith (1991, 1992) particularly wanted to show that emotional labour *needs* to be taught to students because of the public's perception of nurses as intrinsically caring and nurturing, which implies that the ability to meet personal emotional needs is an inherent characteristic of those who choose to nurse.

This chapter examines the work of those who have applied Hochschild's ideas to the nursing profession. How these ideas have been applied is reflected through Vignette 2 'Alix's dad' and Vignette 1 'Half measures'. Throughout the chapter, areas where Hochschild's work does not readily apply to nursing and what impact this might have in how emotional labour in nursing is understood are considered.

Image and identity in nurses and nursing

Multiple images of nurses are presented in television programmes such as *Casualty, Holby City, No Angels, ER, Doctors* and many more. Nurses are often portrayed as the keepers and carers of emotional needs. As the story unfurls, the viewer sees the traumatic history of each 'patient' coming in, in need of expert care. The doctors ably provide medical expertise, and the nurse, with a few aptly chosen words, provides comfort and clarity of insight to her patients' problems without them needing to give her the information that we the viewer are privy to. Through telepathy they know exactly what their patients' issues are, and being emotionally able, know exactly the right words to say, the degree of comfort required and with astonishing insight bring clarity to an otherwise impossible situation. Of course, this is drama rather than real life, but it acts out an image of nursing and nurses that the public needs to believe in. Nurses are seen as being kind, considerate, patient; they are cheerful, loving, friendly, good listeners and empathetic. Smith (1992: 16) quotes a patient as saying that nurses 'relieve pain and suffering not by medical means but by compassion'. Nurses care: this is fundamental to public belief in them. It is part of their image, their identity. However, Smith notes that while 'caring is clearly identified as what nurses do, more importantly it is underpinned by the assumption that caring *fulfils* nurses' desire to be of *service* to others' (Smith 1992: 21, original emphasis).

Smith (1992) suggests that the image of nurses 'born to nurse' is essential to the profession in recruiting and selecting potential students. Candidates who demonstrate a friendly and caring attitude, motivation to actively work with people and whose past experience suggest they are 'naturally predisposed' to be caring, are actively selected. Throughout nurse training, this expression of self-identity is moulded and developed into that of the professional, dedicated nurse, just as Hochschild's flight attendants are moulded into portraying the airline company's image through their physical appearance and emotional labour.

Although there are many other images of nurses (for example, the sex kitten and the battleaxe matron), the image of the girl born to nurse, devoted to caring for the sick, has remained central to nursing since its origins in Florence Nightingale, the 'lady with the lamp'. This representation of nursing was deliberately promoted, in order to combat Dickensian-like caricatures of nurses as ignorant, middle-aged, drunken charwomen of loose morals, so that nursing could be seen as a respectable profession for middle-class women (Huxley 1975; Maggs 1980). The image of the nurse as vocational, altruistic and inherently caring has become known as the 'Nightingale Ethic'. Maggs (1980) suggests that the Nightingale Ethic has become representative of how nurses are supposed to act and behave:

> that is, [it] represent[s] attempts, deliberate and non-deliberate, to erect a model of behaviour, expectations and performance to which all nurses could aspire and subscribe, but [it] also form[s] the basis of the criteria by which nurses and nursing might be judged.
>
> (Maggs 1980: 20)

This is the image of nurses portrayed in television programmes. Characters who do not represent this image are understood to be deviating from the norm. Bone (2002) notes that most of the emotion work carried out by nurses is often invisible; when it is not carried out, however, it becomes more visible, representing something which nurses can be judged for not doing. Much of the literature consequently comments on how emotional labour in nursing is becoming marginalised, unimportant and constrained in response to concerns that it is not being carried out.

Image and identity in 'Alix's dad' (Vignette 2)

The beginning of Vignette 2 is taken from an audio diary by Amelia, an experienced senior staff nurse, followed by an extract from her interview expanding her feelings about the attitudes of Alix's parents. Alix, who was the actual patient, was 19 years old and had suffered a severe head injury due to a road traffic accident. He was unable to communicate or do anything for himself. He required total care. He was cared for on Ward B for over two months. This vignette illustrates how the idea of nurses as caring and empathetic is being contravened.

Alix had been a healthy, young, independent man on the cusp of life. Now he is unable to do anything at all. His parents are understandably distraught. Yet here the nurse seems unable to recognise the awfulness of their situation. She manages her own emotions, using surface acting, in her interaction with the father, but she shows no real concern. It is easy to judge her and see her as lacking in understanding and empathy. Nurses, after all, are supposed to be able to know how to carry out such care and know how to deal with such situations. Nurses should know how to relieve the suffering of these parents with a caring attitude and a few appropriately chosen words.

Because Amelia does not demonstrate an altruistic, caring attitude, her emotional labour could be considered to be deficient, the lack of it making it more visible. This is a little harsh. After all, Alix's father is rude and offensive to her and Pippa (a health care assistant). Nurses are often confronted with difficult and demanding patients and relatives. They are specifically taught how to help them. This is something that Smith (1992) particularly emphasises. Emotional labour is something that *needs* to be taught. The need for this nurse to know how to deal with this situation is evident here. She is polite, however, and takes the father's attitude without comment to him. In effect, Amelia carries out effective surface acting in her emotional labour. There are several resonances here with what Hochschild observed among flight attendants, who were expected to take the abuse of their customers.

This family find themselves in a situation that is beyond the cure of a few kindly meant words and a caring attitude. Emotional labour is an important *part* of nursing, but its value often extends beyond each immediate interaction; it is more than the surface and deep acting of each individual nurse in one moment of time. It is part of a *collaborative* and *therapeutic relationship* built up between nurse and patient – or in this case between the nurse and the relative. This is where emotional labour in nursing differs from what Hochschild observed among flight attendants. Neither the nurse nor the patient and relative is a passive participant in the emotional exchange. In addition, the care needs of this patient and his family are both complex and long term.

However, the interview with Amelia took place two months on from her initial meeting with Alix and his parents described in the extract from her diary. There is still no real evidence in the interview of a collaborative and therapeutic relationship between them. Instead Amelia describes how their behaviour towards her makes her feel. What she has to say is important. Throughout the rest of this chapter, the significance of this is considered.

Feeling rules

Davies (1995) points out that the value and importance of the nurse's image to nursing goes far beyond that of image. It is central to the way in which nurses are given permission by other members of society to care for their intimate needs. Essentially, the process of nursing care involves one perfect stranger carrying out intimate physical, psychological and social care acts with another perfect stranger, with this often taking place in a public place, such as a hospital. In private life, the only people normally this intimate with them would be family members, lovers and/or partners. Yet in health care, patients allow the nurse to care for their physical body, tell her their problems and share details about their personal and private lives. The idea of nurses, who care for and about others as an expression of their identity, is a belief that is needed by patients, because it enables and facilitates intimate acts of care.

Lupton (1996) suggests that this belief is connected with how people see and feel about their physical bodies. She writes:

> Because we understand our bodies as reflecting ourselves, and because certain parts of the body are invested with secrecy and shame, the relationship between the carer and the person cared for differs from other relationships. To care for someone in that way is to express a love and acceptance of sorts, but it is also to exert a degree of power over the

person who is cared for. Caring may be understood as a gift, an action that requires something in return from the person who is cared for, thereby establishing an imbalance of power (Fox 1993, 1995). In the familial caring relationship, the efforts exerted by the carer may be expected to be rewarded with gratitude, love and affection but never by monetary rewards.

(Lupton 1996: 165)

Lupton suggests that an emotional exchange between people occurs when there is physical intimacy. For example, when a family member requires looking after, due to ill health, they become vulnerable to those who care for them. However, this can be mediated through the emotions that each is considered to offer the other in this situation. The carer shows love to the person being cared for, and in return the cared for rewards them with gratitude and love. Bolton (2000) suggests that the emotional labour of nurses is not in fact emotional labour as coined by Hochschild, rather it is emotion work, which the nurses offer to their patients as a gift. She does not see it as an exchange: 'The emotion work nurses offer to patients is given with little or no expectation of a return of their investment – other than the satisfaction they derive from being able to "make a difference"' (Bolton 2000: 584). However, Bolton underestimates the significance of satisfaction nurses receive as a result of their work, and therefore ignores the importance of the gratitude they receive from their patients. The exchange that takes place between nurses and patients reflects Hochschild's (1983) notion of feeling rules, where people manage their emotions by understanding and recognising the degree of emotion they owe to one another (see Chapter 1). In the feeling rules governing care in private relationships, Lupton (1996) identifies the importance that the emotional exchange is freely given – like a gift – in that neither person is given money in exchange for care. The nurse gives emotional care, the patient or relative, gratitude. However, there is an imbalance in the degree of the emotion exchange. The patient has the greater need. This is why the carer holds power over the person being cared for: they can withhold their love and affection and/or take physical or emotional advantage of them. This is where the Nightingale Ethic has an importance greater than that of image. Believing that nurses are intrinsically kind and considerate, and genuinely concerned with the health and wellbeing of their patients, mimics the freely given exchange which takes place in private relationships. It suggests that the vulnerable public can trust the nurse who has power over them, to care.

The role of emotional labour in nursing is an essential part of the exchange between the individual being cared for and the carer. Feeling rules based on the ideal of nurses as being naturally caring operate as 'moral' guidelines by which the patient allows the nurse to care for their intimate physical body, and by which they can impart personal and private information about their feelings, thoughts and way of life. Such a relationship, usually part of intimate private family life, is reproduced in nursing care and is a crucial component of nurses' emotional labour. Nurses' emotional labour, therefore, is different from that of flight attendants in several ways. First, the feeling rules governing exchanges between nurse and patient are more indicative of private emotion work than consumer-orientated emotional labour because not only are they founded on the basis of a freely given gift, but also this freely give gift is governed by feeling rules where each individual understands what emotion is 'owed'. Second, the balance of power between carers and cared for is negotiated through this freely given emotional exchange. Third, in contrast to Hochschild's flight attendants whose emotional labour is carefully controlled and scripted, and whose own emotions are made irrelevant, emotional labour in nursing is an *exchange*. It involves *interactive* processes based on a *relationship* between the nurse and the patient. Neither the nurse nor patient is a passive participant. The emotions of each contribute to the exchange and are predicated on the kind of relationship they have.

Feeling rules in 'Alix's dad' (Vignette 2)

Alix's parents have lost their son. In his place is a person who physically resembles him but is unable to communicate, remember, share or interact with them in any way. Moreover, the care they could be offering is mostly being undertaken by the nurses who are looking after his every physical need. In a sense they are not free to give the gift of care to their son.

The nurses care for Alix's intimate physical needs. He cannot move, talk, wash, dress, sit up, eat, comb his hair, go to the toilet; he is totally dependent on them for his every need. They have complete power over him; if they do not give this care, Alix can do nothing about it. Although he is their patient, he cannot express gratitude to them and the nurses cannot find out what he is thinking or feeling. Despite his incapacity, the nurses felt that they were building up a rapport with him. They noted every blink or twitch or possible expression that might indicate a response. They encouraged his parents to bring in his own clothes, play his favourite music and talk to him as if he could respond.

When Amelia first meets the parents, she gives them an account of the care she has given and apologises for having to dress Alix in a hospital pyjama top rather than his own T-shirt. This is an expression of concern, an acknowledgement that they might prefer to see Alix in something familiar and personal. In Amelia's eyes she was expressing care and forethought towards both Alix and his parents. In return, Amelia expected an acknowledgement of her care. Instead, the father is angry, rude and accusing towards her. He unconsciously breaks the

---

emotion exchange in the feeling rules governing emotional labour. More, he questions the degree of her care. Amelia is indignant and upset at this treatment, compounded by the fact that it continued throughout Alix's stay on the ward. Amelia's response to the father's attitude changes into a hostile one. She believes that Alix's dad is so rude that he is unable to develop a collaborative relationship with the nursing staff. To emphasise her point she uses the counter-example of Ben, whose parents did cooperate.

By constantly challenging the care Amelia gives his son, Alix's father not only fails to offer gratitude, but also deprives her of a sense of satisfaction in the care that she is giving. This makes her defensive and angry. She notes that when 'people are aggressive, watching everything you do and criticising everything you do, and writing down everything, then you don't go in there. You just don't go in there and try and build up a rapport with people'.

Because emotional labour in nursing is an exchange, it requires a response from the recipient; that response needs to acknowledge the nature of the emotional gift the nurse gives through her care. Nurses do hold power. Amelia exercises hers by withholding emotional labour that is part of a collaborative, therapeutic exchange.

Amelia is not oblivious to the family's pain and suffering, however. She says: 'You try and put yourself in their position, and it *is* terrible what is happening'. But this is not, in her eyes, a sufficient excuse for Alix's dad's aggressive attitude.

The question that needs asking here, is what is happening to the relationship between nurses and those they care for, that in this situation, Amelia holds Alix's dad so accountable for his anger and rudeness when she can understand why he might behave like this?

Emotion work and emotional labour: private–public realm

When they begin their training, first year student nurses are often asked to consider the difference between the care of professional, qualified nurses, health care assistants and family members. The students usually identify the importance of being registered nurses, professionally accountable to the NMC Code of Conduct, they note that qualified nurses are knowledgeable carers who understand the different physiological illnesses of their patients and have expert clinical skills. Occasionally, a student who used to be a HCA argues that there is no difference. Few make the suggestion that registered nurses earn more than HCAs, who earn more than the family carers, who earn nothing at all. This is because economic differences between these groups are seldom identified as being relevant to the *meaning* of care. The fact that nurses are paid a salary is often ignored or downplayed. One of the ways patients emotionally reward nurses is by acknowledging that they deserve to be paid more! In the UK this is accepted because the patient does not pay the nurse or Health Care Trust directly. The National Health Service is paid for through taxation, which both the patient *and* the nurse (and all health care professionals) pay. This is distinctly different from the airline industry, where the type of ticket purchased, such as budget, standard or first class, is indicative of the type and degree of service expected by the customer. Although nurses are paid a financial reward, this is perceived as less important than their motivation to nurse because they care; thus, their care is perceived as genuine because their patients matter to them. In this way it is arguable that the meaning of care is linked to personal identity. Thus, the feeling rules involved are similar to ideal types underpinning social values and how individuals personally relate to those values. This is not to suggest that nurses have no financial motives; like others they have material needs and these are strongly motivating. Equally, it does not suggest that caring in this sense is the *only* value inherent in nursing which elicits satisfaction and motivates the nurse. Rather, it suggests that it is an important and underpinning ideal type through which both nurses and society defines, understands and judges the meaning of care and actions relating to it. This is what Maggs (1980) refers to when he notes that the Nightingale Ethic is prescriptive, and represents the way in which both the public and nurses themselves understand and judge their role. Emotional labour is representative of nurses' desire to care and is something that is considered to be freely given. When this feeling rule is challenged, it has significant consequences to the nature of emotional labour given by the nurses, and it impacts on how emotional labour in nursing is understood.

That this feeling rule is being challenged is evident in much of the literature on emotional labour in nursing. With the advent of the Patients' Charter (Department of Health (DoH) 1995), customer complaints and quasi-market principles introduced in the 1990s, the introduction of patient choice, and an increase in a multitude of health care service providers in the private sector (*The NHS Plan*: DoH 2000), there is a cultural trend towards a more consumer-orientated approach. Here, the customer-cum-patient is perceived as having buying power and the right to make demands of those selling the service or product. Bone (2002), writing about nurses' emotional labour in the United States, notes that there is an increasing demand for emotion work as a commodity, found in customer/patient questionnaires (and complaints). Bolton (2001: 93) also suggests that present-day nurses 'have to present a smiling face to patients who now behave as demanding customers and whose expectations of a quality service have been raised beyond anything the current National Health Service could ever hope to offer'. She argues that nurses have become 'emotional jugglers', able to 'calibrate their performances according to the frame of action, choosing whether to match feeling with face' (Bolton 2001: 97). By demanding emotional labour from nurses, patients are fundamentally changing the feeling rules of exchange that have

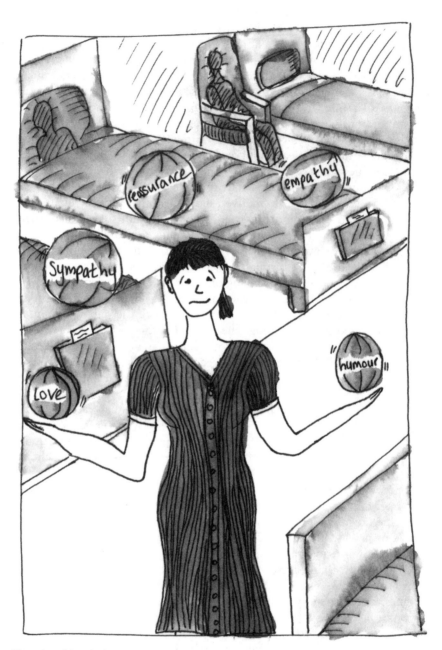

'Emotional juggler'

hitherto mediated the emotional labour process. When this happens, it challenges the belief that the nurse is caring because she is expressing something that is intrinsic to her fundamental character, freely offering care to her patient in exchange for gratitude and personal satisfaction. In addition, the significance of feeling rules that mediate issues of intimacy between nurses and patients by imitating personal and private relationships from the private realm is also lost. This changes the character of the interaction between nurse and patient, and as Bolton (2001) identifies, the emotional labour offered by the nurse becomes much more cursory and surface in nature.

Both Bone (2002) and Bolton (2001) represent nurses' emotional labour or work as a commodity. Hochschild (1983) argues that where emotional labour has commodity value and is controlled by the company for whom the labourer works, a division between the 'real/true self' and the 'false self' is created. This has consequences for what the individual, and society as a whole, perceives as being authentic emotion. Bolton's research reflects this; she quotes a ward sister saying:

> One minute I am smiling politely, one minute I'm crying or trying not to cry, the next minute I'm having a good laugh. I should have been on the stage. I present so many faces through the course of the day it's like being a one-woman stage show.
>
> (Bolton 2001: 97)

This quotation represents a different understanding of the emotional labour exchange. It is one where the sister implies that her presentation of self does not belong to her. Who she is as a person is not present in the interactions she has with her patients. Instead her actions are scripted and performed. Her emotional labour is inauthentic. In Hochschild's work, inauthenticity was experienced by the flight attendants for two main reasons. First, when private emotion work was transmuted into emotional labour as a commodity, what the flight attendants felt, why they should feel it and how they should manage and express it, was dictated and prescribed. Second, the flight attendants became unable to give affective emotional labour when speed-up occurred, compromising, to varying degrees, their perceptions of their identity. In nursing, it appears that inauthenticity is also occurring because nurse's private emotion work has undergone transmutation, becoming a commodity. However, in addition to emotional labour being representative of an emotional exchange, there is a fundamental difference between the emotional labour of nurses and that of flight attendants. That is, as the purveyors of health care, nurses hold power over their patients, whereas flight attendants are vulnerable to the consumer power of their customers.

Emotion work and emotional labour: private–public realm in 'Alix's dad' (Vignette 2)

On the surface, Alix's dad does not demand emotional labour as if it were a commodity. However, he acts as if it is acceptable to treat Amelia (and the other nurses) without respect. Underlying this behaviour is the implication that he has the right to do so. In effect, he demands from Amelia emotional understanding that she had in the first instance offered freely. Amelia implies this by making reference to other patients and their relatives who watch her every move and even write things down. This is an act of aggression, an assertion of power being made by the patient or relatives that says, 'If you do not carry out your work to our satisfaction we will lodge an official complaint, evidenced through our documented observations of your actions'. Amelia interprets Alix's dad's hostility in this way. He broke the relational emotional exchange and demanded professionalism from her in the face of his hostile behaviour. This changed the character of the interaction between him and Amelia; consequently, the emotional labour she offers is cursory and surface in nature. She gives him exactly what he demands but withholds genuine care that seeks to understand his pain and offer comfort to him. As noted earlier, this can seem as if the nurse is uncaring. Because the emotional labour that is offered is indicative of surface acting, it can also seem that the nurse has become inauthentic to herself, smiling and being polite in the face of someone she openly admits she does not like.

The feeling rules which mediate the relationship between nurse and patient or relative by taking private emotion work into the public realm as if it was being undertaken in the private realm, has become emotional labour, a commodity undertaken entirely in the workplace.

Trust and power in emotional labour

In Lupton's (1996) argument, the balance of power between the carer and the cared for lies with the carer because they can withhold care, or abuse the vulnerable position of the cared for. However, in health care, the balance of power between the health care professional and the patient is redressed because the 'nurse–patient relationship is based on reciprocality and exchange. Trust is required on both sides' (Lupton 1996: 165). The reciprocal nature is achieved in the emotion exchange (care is given by the nurse and gratitude is given by the patient), not in the emotional labour process. The nurse does not make herself emotionally vulnerable to her patient; rather she withholds her personal feelings and thoughts using her emotional labour to listen and care, offering advice and comfort to the patient. This is what Davies (1995) refers to when she suggests that emotional labour is important to nursing care because it crosses over the physical and emotional boundaries of what is considered to be private and personal by carrying them out in public. Thus, the Nightingale Ethic is something that nurses can be judged by not only because it represents the permission given by society to nurses to carry out intimate acts of care on their behalf, but also because it suggests that society can trust that the care given to them is in their best interests. Feeling rules pertinent to the emotional labour of nursing therefore centre around alleviating shame and embarrassment related to bodily functions; the safe expression of pain, anger, fear, anxiety and bewilderment related to physical, psychological and emotional concerns; and with the expressions of the nurses' emotions through their labour being ones of humour, empathy, sympathy, love and reassurance. Thus, during nursing training, students are taught how to emotionally respond when presented with a bedpan full of steaming faeces, or how to deal with the 'difficult' patient, or how best to anticipate and respond to patients' anger and grief. Emotional labour helps redress the balance of power held by health care professionals over those who are vulnerable and sick. Patients discuss their personal problems with nurses (and other health care professionals) not just to share them but also because their need is real. They need to trust that the nurse has the expertise to give appropriate care and advice. It is fundamentally important when understanding emotional labour in health care not to underestimate the dependency that sick and vulnerable people have on their carers. The social values encapsulated in the Nightingale Ethic are essential to many of the interactions undertaken in health care because the belief that doctors and nurses act to save and preserve life is fundamental to society having the confidence to accept the care offered. Smith (1992: 3) illustrates this very well when she quotes from a Macmillan nurse recruitment advert: 'Mummy said she had cancer. Daddy got very upset. The nurse made them both feel better.'

Underpinning this is another equally important feeling rule and social value encapsulated within the ideal of a 'pure relationship' (Giddens 1990, 1992). The ability and luxury to communicate freely and honestly with loved ones represents a belief about what constitutes a good relationship. 'Confessing' intimate and personal details to one another (Foucault 1978) creates mutual vulnerability. This is considered to be essential in developing relationships built on trust. It is also representative of a social belief that opening up and talking about personal problems and emotional concerns is beneficial to health and wellbeing. Phrases such as 'a problem shared is a problem halved' imply that talking about problems to someone, such as a counsellor, is therapeutic.

Wouters (1991) suggests that the expression of emotions is related to positioning within social hierarchies. The more hierarchical the organisation (from the NHS to the family), the more important the ability to suppress emotion is in establishing position within it. This is because those with a higher status also have greater power. For example, in Chapter 1 the example of Johnny learning to control his feelings was used. As a young boy he has more licence than an older person to express his emotions. If an adult throws a tantrum when they do not get what they want, or shouts at a child, their behaviour would be frowned on. This hierarchy is replicated in institutions: in health care it is the health care professionals who are expected to manage their emotion, while patients are allowed the freedom to express theirs. However, the current consumer-orientated approach within the NHS has resulted in a shift in the balance of power between carer and patient. 'The "culture of the customer" bestows a superior status to the consumer and the interaction between service provider and customer is an unequal exchange' (Bolton and Boyd 2003: 304). As professionals, nurses are still expected to manage their emotions; however, their power has been reduced as they have become vulnerable to patient complaints.

Hochschild (1983) particularly emphasises how flight attendants are exploited not only through the transmutation of their emotion work but also because in the capitalist system, they are vulnerable to losing their jobs if they do not conform; thus they have limited power. This is not the case in nursing, not because emotional labour is not monitored, nor because nurses are invulnerable to their patient's power to complain about them; it is because the people for whom they care are ill and vulnerable themselves. Their needs are real and their options are often limited. Despite the introduction of quasi-market principles and consumer choice, health and illness are not necessarily accountable to market forces, they cannot always be bought. Emotional labour in nursing therefore is different from that of flight attendants in two ways: first, it involves an interactive emotional exchange, and second, it involves trust, which is crucial to mediating the power and influence that nurses have in their interaction with patients.

Trust and power in emotional labour in 'Alix's dad' (Vignette 2)

A cultural shift concerning the relationship that exists between health care providers and those who require that care has occurred. Bolton and Boyd (2003) suggest that the interaction between service provider and customer in a consumer culture is an unequal exchange because the consumer can exercise their right to question the service that is offered. In health care, this questioning is impacting on the emotional exchange that has traditionally been understood to be freely given. To the nurses it challenges their very integrity. They feel that the quality of their care is being constantly undervalued and undermined. When Amelia mentions to Alix's parents that she and the HCA had, in fact, recently changed Alix despite the fact that he was wet again, she comments 'but they wouldn't believe us, they don't believe you'. Then when the parents, despite contravening the emotional exchange, still expect nurses automatically to know what their patients' needs are without being told, Amelia exclaims indignantly: 'we're not psychic! They seem to think you're psychic as well don't they?'

In Amelia's account, trust and reciprocity in her relationship with Alix's dad, and by inference with other patients and their relatives, has irrevocably broken down. This in turn has impacted on the balance of power between them. It has not affected the giving of emotional labour; that still takes place, albeit on a surface and cursory level. It has, however, fundamentally changed the emotion exchange that takes place. This is a terrible thing. Alix's dad, his hostile attitude not withstanding, is vulnerable and in need. Contravening the feeling rules governing emotional labour by treating the nurse's emotional labour as a commodity has resulted in Amelia withholding her empathy and understanding. But Alix's dad has no choice but to trust in the care that is given to him. In the awfulness of the situation in which he finds himself, he needs to be able to trust in the carers and in the care they give. In his vulnerable state, it is arguable that he is not able to control his anger and resentment. He needs someone who can and is willing to understand this. Amelia is not. As the health care professional with the knowledge and expertise to do this, she exercises her power not to do so. She is not doing this maliciously, however; she is trying to protect herself. She is protecting herself from the power asserted over her through the complaints and the abuse that others now feel free to express. Emotional labour in nursing – as an exchange – involves the interaction of both parties predicated on the relationship they have together. In this case, the relationship has been damaged.

Advancement and speed-up in nursing

Emotional labour is not new to nursing. It is a component of nursing care. Nicky James (1992) suggests that such care involves 'organisation + physical labour + emotional labour'. It is not surprising, therefore, to find that emotional labour is included in the nursing process and in nursing models which take a holistic approach. Holistic care is where the patient's physical, psychological, socio-cultural, politico-economic and spiritual needs are all considered integral to their health and wellbeing. Holistic care depends on both continuity of care and establishing a relationship. This approach makes three fundamental assumptions. The first is that individual nurses will be responsible for the total care of individual patients. Second, that nurses are fully qualified in nursing knowledge and skill to carry out total patient care. Third, that the organisation of nursing work enables both time and continuity of care. This was, arguably, part of the aim behind the introduction of Primary Nursing and the 'Named Nurse' in the Patient's Charter in the 1990s. However, since then there have been significant organisational structural changes, and medical, technological advances in the delivery of health care, impacting on what nursing care is considered to be and how it is carried out.

In 2006 the UK population reached over 60 million, thus demand for health care services has massively risen. However, in the 1990s, centralisation and rationalisation of acute tertiary services, and a shift towards care in the community, reduced the number of hospital beds available. In addition, specific targets to reduce waiting times for health care services introduced under the NHS Plan (DoH 2000) have increased the number of health care procedures performed. All these factors have resulted in fewer resources and greater demand. Thus, the numbers of patients treated has increased while their stay in hospital has been reduced.

In addition, under Project 2000, student nurses became supernumerary to the duty roster. The nursing work they were previously responsible for is now the province of HCAs, who carry out the majority of basic 'hands-on care', while the nurse's role has become more clinical and managerial. As a consequence, a more clearly defined division of labour representative of the available skill mix has impacted on how nursing care is carried out. Under skill mix, the practice of nursing for the trained nurse 'drops through the vacuum in the middle: this is the *polo mint* effect' (Davies 1995: 90). Thus, while the registered nurse is knowledgeable and skilled in carrying out holistic care, this care fails to occur. Instead, patient care is broken down into tasks, devolved and distributed between the different health carers with different skill levels that nurses oversee. Consequently, a division has occurred between what is considered to be basic hands-on care, inclusive of emotional labour, and what is considered clinical and medically technical care. This has had a negative affect on the value ascribed to emotional labour.

For example, Smith (1992) found that first year student nurses valued developing relationships with their patients and carrying out effective emotional labour. However, by the time they entered their final year of training, clinical skills and medical knowledge were given greater status. This attitude has been reinforced with the advances made in medical knowledge and technology. Qualified nurses now take on clinical skills once the province of doctors, in addition to new techniques more recently developed. In fact, a career trajectory in which registered nurses can work towards becoming clinical nurse specialists, managers and nurse consultants has been introduced (DoH 2000). Arguably, this means that the development of nursing practice is the result of the delegation of medical tasks and advances in medical science, the implication being that both traditional hands-on nursing care and nursing knowledge are considered inferior to medically based clinical care (MacKay 1989; Smith 1992; Philips 1996). The role of emotional labour has, therefore, become linked to basic hands-on nursing care. Similarly, emotion is seen as being feminine, and science or reason as being masculine, thus, emotional labour is accorded a lower status than clinically based nursing care. Philips argues that:

> The problem is if we formally acknowledge emotional labour, then the professional standing of the occupation could very well be diminished, primarily because one trait of the classic profession, especially in modern scientific society, is the application of a specialised body of knowledge. It seems the application of emotional labour is unlikely to be regarded as the application of such a body of knowledge.
>
> (Philips 1996: 142)

The value of emotional labour has been undermined by the development and changes in the nurse's role and in the division of labour. This is compounded by the massive increase in the volume and pace of nursing work in the hospital setting. Nicky James (1989, 1992), who investigated emotional labour in hospices, argues that effective emotional labour requires flexibility in the organisational structure. For, 'emotional labour takes time and requires considerable knowledge of the patient as a person' (James 1992: 503). Thus 'even when staff actively seek to give "good patient care"', tensions between 'organisational priorities and organising individual patient care may appear insurmountable' (James 1992: 495). Nurses are exceptionally busy juggling a high volume of work with increasingly shorter patient hospital stays. Thus as Olesen and Bone note:

> Registered nurses intervene with technical skills and oversee and document the work performed by others. They may be responsible for a greater number of patients, but are no longer providing primary care. The overall impact of managed care has been to decrease the number of nurses involved in direct patient care while increasing the levels of responsibility for patient outcome. In general, this has reduced the amount of time available for all aspects of work, including emotional labour.
>
> (Olesen and Bone 1998: 320)

This has had a negative effect on emotional labour in nursing. Bone (2002: 144) argues that 'emotionality expressed in today's market driven health care settings more often reflects emotional dissonance than ideal types of emotional support'. Although Olesen and Bone (1998) and Bone (2002) are referring to the US health care system, the outcome is much the same in the UK. Overall, an increase in the pace and quantity of nursing care, a decrease in the significance given to emotional labour at a time when patients/relatives are demanding it like a commodity is resulting in nurse stress, burnout and inauthenticity of self (Majomi et al. 2003; Montgomery et al. 2006).

Advancement and speed-up in 'Half measures' and 'Alix's dad' (Vignettes 1 and 2)

Issues concerning both advancement and speed-up in nursing are particularly evident in Vignette 1, 'Half measures'. Here, in response to the question about what constitutes good care, Paris answers without hesitation: 'Obviously clinically I would be able to look after my patients properly.' She prioritises the clinical over the psychological and emotional. She also makes a clear demarcation between the clinical and the psychological-cum-emotional component of nursing. She notes that when she was a more junior member of staff, she had more time to carry out such care. This reflects Nicky James' (1992) recognition that good emotional labour requires time, and therefore flexibility in the organisation of nursing work. Now Paris tries to meet the many physical and clinical needs of her patients halfway. While clinical care is clearly prioritised and given greater status, the value and importance of emotional labour is still recognised and Paris still uses it as a measurement of good quality nursing care that elicits satisfaction. Bone (2002) comments that emotional labour represents something that is intrinsic and important yet lost to nursing. She observed that 'the nurses expressed feelings of loss and remembered feelings no longer possible under current working conditions. Grieving the loss of something taken for granted is doubly painful; it must be acknowledged and then released' (Bone 2002: 144). The pain in remembering previous emotional care given, and the inability to make time to do so now, was so painful to Paris that it reduced her to tears on several occasions.

In Vignette 2, 'Alix's dad', there is a slightly different representation of the division of labour in nursing care. Despite Amelia being a senior staff nurse, she carried out basic hands-on care, washing, changing and toileting Alix with Pippa the HCA. While qualified nurses are undoubtedly taking on more clinical and managerial responsibilities – indeed much of their work can be done only because they are registered nurses – this does not equate to them never carrying out basic hands-on care. Equally, Amelia's comments imply that she frequently carried out such care for Alix and other patients. This suggests that the belief that qualified nurses no longer carry out basic hands-on care needs to be questioned. Amelia also suggests that it is not because she has no time to carry out emotional labour; it is the attitudes of the patients and their relatives that inhibit her. This suggests that the way in which emotional labour is carried out is variable and complex. The accounts that Paris and Alix give are different but equally valid.

Emotional labour in nursing

The account given of the condition of emotional labour in nursing is not a positive one. Bolton (2001: 86) summarises its overall representation in the literature as one where it has been 'shown that though emotion work is a vital part of the nursing labour process it tends to be marginalised'. Nurses have become 'accomplished social actors and multi-skilled emotion managers' able to present a variety of faces; 'the professional face, smiley face and humorous face, against the backdrop of structural changes affecting the British public sector services'. Under the cover of these faces, 'nurses are able to manipulate and resist some the emotional demands made of them while still presenting an acceptable face' (Bolton 2001: 86). Emotional labour as an essential component of nursing care, inherent in the therapeutic relationship built between nurse and patient, has evolved into a commodity that results in nurses performing and presenting different faces like puppets on strings.

Thus, like Hochschild's flight attendants, nurses have been shown to have little time to carry out effective emotional labour; to be defensive when emotional labour is demanded from them as a commodity; and their sense of emotional authenticity lost in prescriptive puppet-like emotion expressions. This is distressing because emotional labour is an essential component of the need and purpose of nursing care. It is essential in negotiating the intimate and personal nature of the interactions between nurses and their patients: in mediating the balance of power between nurses and those they care for and in promoting and maintaining trust in people who seek care when they are vulnerable and in need.

The evidence of these changes is apparent in both Vignette 1 and Vignette 2. In Vignette 1, Paris is distraught because she has no time or space in which she can give good nursing care, instead her desire to do so is suppressed, and a professional demeanour is adopted. In Vignette 2, Amelia is defensive about the unreasonable demands made of her. She suppresses her hurt and anger and presents a professional face giving exactly what is demanded, but no more.

This account of emotional labour in nursing is one that the profession needs to address. Nursing still involves face-to-face contact, the needs of the patient are still primary and emotional labour as a part of interpersonal and communication skills is still taught and monitored. That emotional labour is considered to be marginalised is disturbing. However, the application of Hochschild's (1983) notion of emotional labour to nursing is not straightforward. McClure and Murphy (2007: 101) argue that her notion of emotional labour is 'unable to adequately account for the emotionally complex emotional role behaviours and demands of professional nurses'. Significant differences between the emotional labour of nurses to that of Hochschild's flight attendants have been identified in this chapter. These differences are significant and need to be investigated. However,

Hochschild's notion of emotional labour also has immense application and continuing relevancy to nursing. Thus, developing her notion of emotional labour in respect to the differences identified, and then applying it to nursing in order to better understand emotional labour in nursing, is as valuable as finding an alternative approach.

In this chapter, four key differences have been identified. First, emotional labour is an integrated component of holistic nursing care. How it is incorporated and carried out within that role is different to that of flight attendants. Understanding the holistic nature of emotional labour may help in identifying it within nursing practice. Second, emotional labour is part of a collaborative and therapeutic relationship between the nurse and patient. It is an interactive and relational process. In Hochschild's work, emotional labour is seen only from the flight attendant's and the airline company's perspective. It is not seen as an interactive exchange taking place between the flight attendant and the passenger as part of their relationship. Understanding the process of emotional labour in nursing requires some knowledge of the relationship between the recipient and the giver in order to identify its purpose. That relationship may be expressive of the immediate interaction taking place, or it may contribute towards the development of the relationship over a period of time. Third, emotional labour is *needed* by patients because they are vulnerable. Emotional labour in nursing and its accompanying feeling rules are therefore crucial in promoting trust and mediating the balance of power that nurses hold over their patients. Understanding the role of trust and power is vital to understanding emotional labour in nursing. This is different from Hochschild's flight attendants, who are themselves vulnerable and who Hochschild clearly sees as being exploited by both the customers and the airline company. Fourth, as an emotional exchange, emotional labour involves an exchange of *emotions*. Thus, identifying what those emotions are is important to understanding the nature of the emotional labour exchange.

How Hochschild conceptualises emotional labour and the context in which emotional labour is carried out in nursing has been explored. However, the nature of emotion has not yet been considered. Emotional labour is about the management of emotions; it is emotions that are exchanged in the process; it is the power of emotion that can hurt or support. Emotion is a key factor connecting the four differences between the emotional labour of flight attendants and nurses. Each one reflects a facet of emotion. Understanding the relationship between emotional labour and emotion therefore is essential to developing the concept of emotional labour. How Hochschild conceptualises emotion and applies that to emotional labour is examined in Chapters 3 and 4.

Vignette 3 'The scrotal drain'

(From my participant observation diary)

I'm in A & B bay again with Susan [a student nurse who will later feature in Vignette 4]. It has been a really nice shift actually. I gave B bay to Susan as she wants the experience of managing acute patients on her own. Which after making sure she knows what she's doing and where to find me, etc., meant I had just nine patients this morning which was so nice. The best thing was this removal of a drain I did for this 45-year-old gentleman. He was one day post-op, as yesterday he had a surgical 'drainage of a scrotal abscess'. He's a postman actually and he developed this huge abscess in his scrotum from riding on his bike to deliver the mail every day. It's easy to see how it happened, must have been really painful. Anyway, in theatre they put in this corrugated drain to help all the fluid flow out of the wound site post-op. Then today on the doctor's ward round they asked me to take it out. Well, you should have seen the look on his face. I mean this drain isn't small, and while having it put in under anaesthetic is one thing, taking it out without is quite another. There was pretty much a collective gasp from all the other men in the bay and I think all their sympathetic looks made him even more afraid! Anyway, taking this drain out, and repacking the wound for me wouldn't be that difficult, but for this gentleman it was a real ordeal and basically he was terrified. Basically managing his fear was the most important thing because the more tense he was, the more difficult it would have been to take the drain out with him tensing and jumping with every move I made. And what was so great about this was that I had time to do it properly. So first I made sure we had a chat about how I was going to do it and what his options were about pain relief. So I explained that I could give him analgesia 30 minutes before I did the dressing and that if he wanted I could get gas and air up for him to use throughout the procedure. In that way he would have more control over his pain control. Men are such babies when it comes to their private bits and it seemed really appropriate getting him gas and air – which he decided that he definitely wanted – as it's what we give women in childbirth! So anyway, I organised with the porters to bring up some gas and air and I gave him Brufen 30 minutes before-hand and made sure that he knew how to work the gas and air. It was quite amusing really, as when I actually came to do the dressing all the other men in the bay were sat on their beds with their legs firmly crossed in sympathy!! So I drew the curtains round to give him some privacy but knew that all the other men would be listening to what was going on. So I pumped up the bed and laid out my trolley and we started chatting about his son. His son is about eight and they love playing football together and he's a real supporter of the Us, and at the same time I was explaining everything like I was doing.

'I'm just going to clean your wound now, it may feel a bit cold but it shouldn't hurt – so you and your son like to pass the ball . . . how did that feel? Okay . . . Good. So you reckon your son's going to make striker one day? Are you doing okay? No pain? That's good, so maybe he'll get signed to play for the U's?' and then I said, 'How are you doing?' and he said, 'Okay' then I said, 'Well you can relax now because I've already taken it out!' He was so surprised and then all the other men in the bay started to clap, so I put my head round the curtain and gave a curtsey!! Then I finished cleaning up. I was really chuffed. The whole thing went off splendidly.

3   Emotion and cognition

The systematic study of emotions in sociology began only as recently as the 1970s (Turner and Stets 2005). Hochschild was among the first to develop a sociological understanding of emotion. At the time there were two distinct schools of thought on emotion: the organismic school, which focused primarily on the organic, biological and psychological nature of emotion, and the social constructionist school, which saw emotions as constructed and given meaning by people according to their cultural and social ideology. Two important debates divided these schools. The first debate considered whether emotion was rational or irrational. The second debate was on whether emotion was an instinctive response linked to biological, innate survival processes and general bodily function, or whether it was subject to cognition, linked to rational thought processes and therefore manageable. Hochschild, however, is considered to transcend the biology–society divide (S. Williams 1998a). She set out to find the middle ground between organismic and constructionist models by developing the work of interactionist theorists Goffman, Dewey, Gerth, Mills and Mead and applying their approach to Darwin's theory of gesture and Freud's cognitive representation of emotion from the organismic school. In Appendix A of *The Managed Heart*, Hochschild (1983) grapples with these debates and explores these different models and theoretical approaches to emotion, producing a new integrated social theory of emotion. She defines emotion as being like a biological *sense* such as smell or touch which is '*unique* among the senses, because it is related not only to an orientation toward action but also an orientation toward cognition' (Hochschild 1983: 219). Bringing together these different theoretical perspectives she defines her social theory of emotion as being

> what gets 'done to' emotion and how feelings are permeable to what gets done to them. From Darwin, in the organismic tradition, I posit a sense of what is there, impermeable, to be 'done to', namely, a biologically given sense related toward an orientation toward action. Finally through Freud, I circle back from the organismic to the interactional tradition, tracing through an analysis of the signal function of feeling how social factors influence what we expect and thus what feelings 'signal'.
>
> (Hochschild 1983: 222)

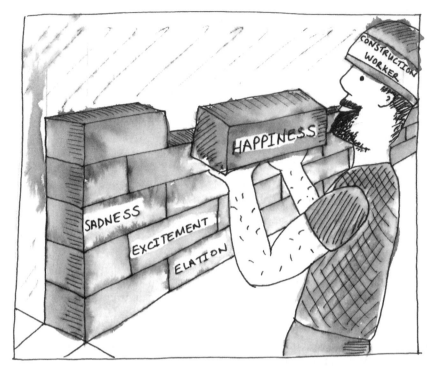

'Emotion constructionist'

Hochschild's approach acknowledges that emotion is not simply a biological entity internally stored and 'outed' on stimulation. *How* feeling is managed can both affect and create emotion as well. Her approach constructs a biopsychosocial understanding of emotion, which has interactionism at its heart, making it fundamentally sociological. This approach towards emotion enabled her to develop her notion of emotion management and emotional labour and therefore underpins them. The purpose of this chapter is to examine how Hochschild (1983) conceptualises emotion in respect to cognition, and to consider how that impacts on her understanding of emotion management/emotional labour. The significance of this is then assessed in respect to the four key differences in the emotional labour of nurses to that of flight attendants identified in Chapter 2 (see Table 3.1).

Emotion: innate and independent or subject to cognition? The linguistic argument

At the beginning of her Appendix A, Hochschild (1983) states that emotion is a suitable concept that can be – and should be – studied independently. It should not however be subsumed into concepts such as cognition or

Table 3.1 Four key differences between the emotional labour of nurses and that of flight attendants

---

- Emotional labour is part of *holistic* nursing care.

- Emotional labour is part of a collaborative, interactive and relational process involved in developing a therapeutic relationship between the nurse and her patient. Emotional labour can be more than the management of emotion in one given moment of time.

- Emotional labour is *needed* by patients because they are vulnerable; emotional labour is therefore implicated in mediating power and trust within the caring relationship.

- Emotional labour involves an emotional exchange. Emotional labour therefore involves an exchange of *emotions*.

---

affect, because in doing so, 'we lose the idea that emotions reflect the individual's sense of the self-relevance of a perceived situation. We lose an appreciation of what the language of emotion can tell us' (Hochschild 1983: 202).

The cognitive approach to emotion emphasises the idea that emotions do not come into being until a judgement about the 'object' or 'social/cultural event' with which the individual finds themselves engaging, has been made. Following the evaluation of the situation, the individual decides whether this will be potentially harmful or beneficial (Strongman 1987; Cornelius 1996; Lazarus 1999; Turner and Stets 2005). The subsequent emotion will reflect this evaluation and help in coping with it (Folkman and Lazarus 1988; Lazarus 1999). For example, if an individual finds themselves in an argument and their opponent insults them, they would make a judgement about the degree of the insult. The resulting emotion, such as indignation (if the insult was moderate) or anger (if the insult was really offensive) would come about after they had evaluated the degree of the insult according to the situation in which it arose and the person delivering it. Previous to that judgement, the emotion would not exist. The difficulty with cognitive appraisal is that the individual's sense of relevance of the situation they find themselves in is lost. The individual actually experiences the emotion immediately, the sensation of indignation or anger, infusing them. The emotion is immediately understandable because of the context in which it arose. Their bodies become flushed and their heart rate increases and it might feel to them as if the emotion is engulfing them rather than it having come into being after evaluating the situation. If emotion is studied from a cognitive perspective only, the relevance of the individual's experience and interpretation of that emotion is lost. Cognition therefore subsumes the experience of emotion rather than the experience of emotion being relevant and illuminating in its own right.

However, the experience of emotion can be understood through language.

> There is a loss when emotion is conceptually ripped away from the situation to which it is attached . . . Just as modern linguists now examine language as it is used in the social context, so emotion, another sort of language, is best understood in relation to its social context.
>
> (Hochschild 1983: 203)

This is because language is used to describe what emotions feel like. Emotions are therefore illustrated as being 'overwhelming' or 'consuming', 'building up', 'being frazzled'. This is an ambitious argument because just as language makes the social context more understandable and can be used to make individual emotion experiences more communicable, it is also the means by which cognitive appraisals are made. Any process that involves making judgements, evaluations or appraisals involves some degree of rational processing, which is mostly understood through language. This is problematic because Hochschild uses language to consider whether emotion can have an independent presence in individuals.

This debate centres on whether emotion can occur in a way that cannot be controlled because it exists independently of free will. Can emotion cause individuals to act by bypassing their cognitive processes? Hochschild argues that the representation of emotion in language makes it seem like it can. For example, emotions may be described as something that can 'strike', 'betray', 'grip', 'paralyze' or 'overwhelm' (Hochschild 1983: 203). Although this use of language suggests emotion is independent of individual will, Hochschild argues that this merely represents the *fiction* of autonomous emotion, in order that the contrast or conflict between inner feeling and outer expressions can be understood. For example, following an insult the resulting anger can overwhelm the individual to such a degree that it can cause them to shout and retaliate almost instantly. In this sense they may experience the anger as betraying inner feelings that they would have preferred to remain hidden, wanting instead to appear cool and indifferent to the insult. Use of such metaphorical language as 'betraying' and 'overwhelming' implies that emotion has *caused the individual to act independently of their will*, suggesting that emotion has its own agency. The apparent agency given to emotion in language describes what it 'feels like' only when experiencing a sudden surge of emotion. However, Hochschild argues that the conclusion that it actually has such autonomy cannot be drawn, because allowing language to define emotion as having individual presence and agency prevents understanding about how emotion actually works. She suggests that since emotion is not independent of our experience of it through its representation in language, it therefore cannot be independent. This is inconsistent because her argument still hinges on what language teaches about the nature of emotion. For, she presents emotion as not being independent even though our experience of it makes it feel like it is. Equally, Hochschild's claim that language does not reveal the nature of emotion appears inconsistent with her previous comment that language helps understand the experience of it.

Hochschild is making a fine distinction here between the *nature* of emotion and the *experience* of emotion. In the end, she appears to agree with the cognitive approach that sees emotion (by its nature) as being subject to cognitive appraisal. But, she also wants to suggest that this is not how individuals may experience it. This is partly because *sociologically*, how individuals interpret, act and respond to the social world around them is encapsulated in language. Language is culturally and socially constructed. In empirical terms, the observation and documentation of social interaction is based on interviews and observation notes; language – which is then interpreted. Hochschild uses language, therefore, in the analysis of her interviews and observations of flight attendants. Thus she analyses their individual representations of their emotion experiences through the language they use. However, her theory develops her understanding of the management of emotion – which is based on the belief that emotion is and can be interpreted and controlled by reason. Thus, Hochschild's notion of emotion management hinges on the continuum between how we experience emotion and how we manage it and the relationship between the two. The whole premise of emotion management itself is based on the belief that emotion is innately manageable. Thus, in her theory of emotion she says it is about 'what gets done to emotion and how feelings are permeable to what gets done to them' (Hochschild 1983: 222). This indicates that emotion is a passive sense waiting for cognition to define and shape its meaning and purpose. Therefore, she renders emotion as dependent on and accountable to cognition.

Emotion and cognition: the linguistic argument in 'The scrotal drain' (Vignette 3)

Vignette 3 is taken from my participant observation notes, documenting my thoughts and feelings about daily life on Ward B. Language is used to describe and explain those feelings.

Vignette 3 is a good example of cognitive appraisal. Prior to the doctor's ward round, the patient was not particularly feeling anxious in any apparent way. On hearing the doctor's request however, his anxiety begins to develop. In the vignette I comment: 'You should have seen the look on his face', noting the visibility of the presence of emotion. This statement assumes that this is a shared judgement about the experience he will be going to have. In fact, there is a shared expectation as the other men take 'a collective gasp' in sympathy. This also affects the postman, confirming his evaluation about the degree of pain he is likely to experience, increasing his anxiety. I also estimate the degree of anxiety, suggesting that he is more than anxious, he is terrified and I talk about managing his 'fear'. Cognitive appraisal has been carried out by the patient, me and the other men in the bay.

Cognitive approaches to emotion suggest that if the situation is judged to be harmful, negative emotions, such as anxiety, will follow, then coping strategies will emerge in order to manage the emotion (Lazarus 1991, 1999). As his nurse, my primary task was to enable my patient to manage his fear. I did this by trying to give him more control of the situation by acknowledging the degree of his anxiety and the degree of pain he was anticipating, and by explaining what I was going to do and what his pain control options were. Giving him this information helped him to re-evaluate his expectation of what would happen. If the nurse understands and has strategies of reducing the ordeal, then it might not be as bad as expected.

Offering him options over his pain relief and in his choice of gas and air gave him control over his pain management. Knowing this also enabled him to re-evaluate his expectation of what would occur during the procedure. In addition, throughout the procedure I chat away on a subject that he is comfortable with and which evokes more happy feelings. This has two effects. First, it diverts his attention towards the conversation in addition to the procedure, and second, my relaxed approach helps his confidence in my abilities because I am implicitly saying there is nothing to worry about and everything is fine, without ignoring or dismissing his concerns.

It seems that a cognitive approach to emotion has enabled the identification of the emotion anxiety and an evaluation of its degree (anxiety – fear – terror) and facilitated understanding how it was managed through the analysis of this textual representation of the event.

However, underpinning my emotional labour is the belief that his anxiety will impact on his physical body – causing him to tense and jump around in an uncontrollable way that might bypass his ability to manage his body's physical emotion response. This would make both the clinical task more difficult to carry out, and his pain and distress more acute.

Emotion: independent from or subject to cognition? The biological approach

Understanding how emotion is experienced through its representation in language is a good argument. Empirically it is also necessary. The use of language demonstrates that emotion is linked with, and understood through, cognitive processes. The difficulty with Hochschild's attempt is her use of language as evidence for whether emotion is independent of cognition. To assess the independence of emotion from cognition it is necessary to engage with the biological (or organismic) paradigm. In her Appendix A, Hochschild

(1983) does so, but in a limited way. She assumes that she has already dealt with whether emotion can be independent from cognition through her argument about its representation in language. Therefore, she does not go on to engage with organismic theories about the nature of emotion. Instead, she makes an assumption that emotion always 'signals' or is stimulated by *external* social factors or psychological factors that require cognitive awareness (Hochschild 1983: 221–222). This is problematic in two ways.

First, experiencing emotion as a result of an external trigger does not mean that emotion is absent prior to the stimulus. For example, using Hochschild's own definition of emotion as a sense, the sense of taste is triggered when an individual eats ice cream. The ice cream has an independent and objective presence before they decide to eat it. Their sense of taste is also independently present. This is known because if taste buds are destroyed (through radiation for example) no matter how much the individual attempts to trigger their sense of taste by stimulating it with ice cream they could not, because their taste buds would be absent. Similarly, if the amygdala in the brain is damaged, it limits the ability to experience emotion. Second, it assumes that individuals are *always* cognitively aware of the stimulus. This assumption is based on Hochschild's understanding of cognition. In her discussion of Freud and her evaluation of what elements of cognition to use, she does not define what cognition is, or differentiate between conscious, pre-conscious and unconscious aspects of cognition. The difficulty with this is that if understanding about emotion is based on thought processes that are always discernable it renders the field of psychology and psychoanalysis (and the notion of the unconscious) redundant (Bowers 1984; LeDoux 1998). In suggesting that emotion is not present independently of cognitive awareness, Hochschild effectively says that emotion is synthesised through cognition, making cognition the stimulus. This is similar to clinical psychological positions, which suggest that 'cognitive appraisal (of meaning or significance) underlies and is an integral feature of *all* emotion states' (Lazarus 1982: 1021, original emphasis).

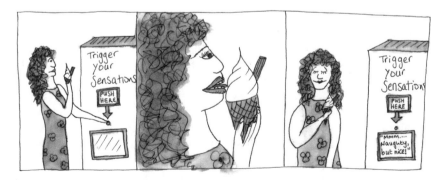

'Cognition ice cream'

Within the organismic school, especially within neuroscience, this is hotly disputed. Zajonc (1984: 118) for example argues that emotion does not need 'cognitive appraisal as a necessary precondition'. Substantial neuro-scientific evidence supports this claim. The evolutionary development of the origin of affect before cognition suggests its primacy (Izard 1984). The identification of separate neuro-anatomical structures for emotion and for cognition (Schwartz et al. 1975; Cacioppo and Petty 1981) provides support-ing evidence. In addition, if cognition is necessary for emotion experience then it should result in cognition *always* changing or controlling emotion, which is not *always* the case (Zajonc 1984).

Understanding how emotions emerge and are activated in the brain has since been substantially developed:

> Emotions emerge as the brain activates four body systems: the auto-nomic nervous system, the neurotransmitter and neuroactive peptide systems, the more inclusive hormonal system and the musculoskeletal system, which interacts with all of the other systems to generate observ-able emotional responses (LeDoux 1996, Turner 2000). These systems are *more than passive motors* that are driven by culture and social structure. They are engines that *have independent effects* on the arousal and expression of emotions.
>
> (Turner and Stets 2005: 4, my emphasis)

Scientific experiments have found that there is a pathway from the retina to the hypothalamus, provoking a direct emotion response based on sensory input from the eye. Emotions that arise like this can bypass cognitive pathways entirely. It is on this physiological principle that the flight/fight reaction operates (Zajonc 1984; LeDoux 1998). 'No mediation by higher mental processes is apparently required. Emotions could be only one synapse away. It is possible that rapidly changing light gradients, such as those that arise with looming objects, could generate fear reactions directly' (Zajonc 1984: 119). For example, developing William James' (1884) 'Feedback Theory', LeDoux (1996, 1998) explains how the body reacts and acts before cognitive processes make the person consciously aware of the threat they are running from. If a grizzly bear suddenly materialises behind a person, their eye detects a change in the light gradient and their ears hear its approach; these sensory messages go straight to the thalamus, which signals to both the subcortical area and the neocortex. The subcortical area is nearer to the thalamus than the neocortex. This results in the immediate stimulation of the autonomic nervous system: the heart pounds, blood pressure rises, the body sweats, and in the immediate stimulation of the musculoskeletal system causing the person to run *before* the message reaches the neocortex and they become consciously aware that it is a bear they are running from (James 1884; LeDoux 1998; Turner and Stets 2005). Evidence indicates therefore that emotion can bypass cognitive processes, suggesting that emotion can be independent and autonomous from cognition.

Hochschild did not engage with this understanding of emotion. However, neuroscientific understanding of emotion has substantially developed since she published *The Managed Heart* in 1983. It is important, therefore, to consider its sociological relevance. First, neuroscientific understanding is relevant when emotional labour is applied to the health care context. In health care the biomedical model has primacy, thus the majority of health care interventions are predicated on biomedical knowledge. Consequently, the management of emotion in nursing includes managing its biological-physical nature. Neuroscience suggests that anxiety and fear do not always lend themselves to being consciously managed. Drug therapy is typically used to depress or switch off the physiological activity causing the anxiety in these incidences. Emotional labour in nursing therefore incorporates a biomedical approach based on neuroscience.

Second, if the mechanism that exists for emotion to cause action independently from cognition is considered, it is possible that emotion may also influence cognition. This is sociologically significant to understanding how emotion is managed, when that management is based on cognitive ability. If it is possible that emotion can bypass cognitive approaches then it may also *influence* cognition. Because Hochschild argues that emotion is orientated towards action mediated through rational management of emotion itself, she does not allow for the possibility that emotion can influence cognitive processes, or socially and culturally motivate apparently irrational acts. Archer (2000), however, suggests that:

> Cognitivists who maintain that our emotions derive from our cognitive interpretations imposed upon reality, rather than from reality itself, have the problems a) of explaining where any commitment (such as becoming a 'concert pianist') comes from if emotions provide no shoving power, b) how they can be maintained without (in this case) positive feedback from practical reality signalling (some) performative achievement, and, c) how, since negative feedback in the form of incompetence would lead to modified career aspirations, we can disregard encounters with reality and view all of them as sieved through some pre-existent and utterly resilient cognitive focus. Instead, emotions are like any other emergent property in that one of their powers *qua* emergents is to modify those of its constituents – in this case the cognitive goal itself.
>
> (Archer 2000: 196)

Knowing we are good at something brings an emotional reward; that reward can become a motivator in itself – thus emotion can influence cognitive choices.

It seems that Hochschild's approach towards the relationship between cognition and emotion can limit understanding of the nature of emotion and its impact on emotional labour. This is not to suggest that Hochschild has it all wrong. Chapters one and two demonstrate clearly that emotion can be, and often is, subject to rational processes of management and defined and understood through socially and culturally based feeling rules, norms and values. Rather, with increased neuroscientific understanding of emotion, it is no longer possible for social scientists to ignore its relevance: 'emotions are generated through systems of interconnected pathways within and between subcortical and neocortical regions of the brain' and 'emotional arousal from various regions of the subcortex is routed through the amygdala to the prefrontal cortex, which is the front portion of the neocortex responsible for rational thought, planning and control of emotions' (Turner and Stets 2005: 7).

Accepting that the relationship between emotion and cognition is complex and interdependent is necessary. It can be the case therefore, that emotion may sometimes override cognition and vice versa, and may sometimes work together.

Emotion and cognition: the biological approach in 'The scrotal drain' (Vignette 3)

In Vignette 3, an important part of my motivation in managing my patient's fear was because 'the more tense he was, the more difficult it would have been to take the drain out with his tensing and jumping with every move I made'. This comment recognises that it is not always possible to will the body into submission. Sometimes it reacts regardless. Anxiety is part of the flight/fight response to the anticipation of a threat. In this case the anticipated threat was pain. When the body goes into flight/fight mode physiological changes take place, the 'blood pressure rises, heart rate increases, pupils dilate, palms sweat, muscles contract in certain ways' (LeDoux 1998: 44). Not all of these changes are outwardly visible. Individuals may believe or claim that they are in control of their emotion responses, but their bodies may react nonetheless. In health care, the body's physiological responses are closely monitored, and these reactions are taken into consideration. When muscles contract (or tense) they either become ready to take off in an instance, or to strike out; anxiety, therefore, can cause the patient to tense and jump, making the nursing procedure much more difficult to carry out. Muscles are very receptive to stimuli, so touching – in cleaning and removing the drain – can cause the patient to jump and twitch in a way that is very difficult to control, increasing his pain and discomfort.

Controlling this response included giving analgesic drugs. This is because the anxiety is elicited in response to anticipated pain. The drugs chosen in this case were gas and air and Brufen. Brufen is a nonsteroidal anti-inflammatory drug which blocks Cox enzymes involved in producing prostaglandins which promote pain and inflammation. Emotion management in nursing involves identifying what emotions are being elicited and what they are being elicited in response to. Some of those responses will be biological. This is considered to affect the emotion management process. Hochschild's understanding of emotion does not adequately account for this.

In addition to anxiety, the emotion of satisfaction is also apparent in the vignette: my satisfaction in a job well done and pride that others witnessed and valued that. The performative achievement in removing the drain without causing the postman any degree of pain was satisfying. In addition, no doubt or concern is expressed over my ability to remove the drain, suggesting previous experiences of satisfaction as a result of competent clinical skills. Thus, confidence and the expectation of satisfaction provided 'shoving power' to how I chose to carry out the task at hand.

Conclusion

At the beginning of her Appendix A, Hochschild (1983) makes the assertion that emotion should not be subsumed into cognition because in doing so its individuation is lost. This assertion loses its value because a full engagement with neuroscientific evidence about the relationship between emotion and cognition is not made. Instead, Hochschild uses the linguistic argument, allowing her to empirically examine the experience of emotion while retaining the primacy of cognition. However, if emotion is subject to cognition and therefore rational by nature, it loses its individuation. As Archer (2000) notes, such an approach does not allow any room for emotion to impact on processes of cognition, nor does it allow room for its spontaneous expression or for it to powerfully motivate apparently irrational action, or simply to be unpredictable or unknowable. Equally, it begs the question if emotion is not independent from cognition in any way, why is it necessary to manage, induce or suppress it? Consequently, Hochschild's insistence on emotion being dependent on cognition makes it difficult for her own analysis not to become subsumed by cognition. While she attempts to straddle the biology–society divide, she actually falls foul of the criticism that she reduces emotion to socially constructed cognitive appraisal.

In some ways this is an unfair assessment of Hochschild's argument, since she bases it on the experience of emotion in language. On this basis, her evaluation of the relationship between emotion and cognition is reasonable.

Understanding the experience of emotion as represented through language is essential. Equally, cognitive approaches in understanding emotion and emotion management are also essential. However, because Hochschild does not address organismic understandings of the physiological nature of emotion, she does not include vital understandings about its neurological relationship with cognitive process. This compromises how the embodiment of emotion is conceptualised when Hochschild's framework is applied to health and illness (Freund 1990; V. James and Gabe 1996; Bendelow and Williams 1998). In her desire to accept that emotion has a biological nature while retaining the value of exploring the experience of emotion in language it would be better to suggest that both language and physical embodied experiences of emotion inform us about its nature.

> An emotion is produced in discourse to the extent that it is named and described using language. This process of naming and describing serves to interpret a constellation of bodily feelings as a particular 'emotion'. But language is not the only means of constructing and expressing emotion. While it is important to recognise the discursive nature of the emotion, their bodily 'presence' or manifestation is also integral. As de Swaan (1990: 168) has vividly put it in relation to jealousy and envy, they are 'gut feelings', often acute and painful physical sensations, 'stings and pangs' with which the body reacts.
>
> (Lupton 1998: 32)

While denying that language can tell us about the nature of emotion, therefore, Hochschild's new theory of emotion fails to develop two essential characteristics, which impact on how she conceptualises the relationship between emotion and its management. This is evident when the four key differences between the emotional labour of nurses and that of flight attendants in Table 3.1 are reassessed.

First, looking at the capacity of emotion to affect cognitive processes suggests that emotion might influence the individual's emotional labour through its constant dialogue with their sense of self over a period of time. For example, in Vignette 3 'The scrotal drain', it was seen that past emotions – such as satisfaction – elicited as a result of performative achievement influenced the manner in which the emotional labour was carried out. Developing this understanding of the nature of emotion further might illuminate how emotional labour is linked to identity. Equally, by accepting the emotion can override cognition, the physical manifestation of emotion and the holistic approach towards its management in health care can be identified.

Second, evaluating the role of cognitive appraisal and emotion in Vignette 3 revealed that as well as being an individual process, cognitive appraisal was also a shared collective one. The emotion management involved a collaborative and interactive process as part of the therapeutic relationship between the nurse and the patient. Hochschild's approach should enable this analysis, yet in Chapter 2 this was not the case. This suggests that it is important to understand how she incorporates her notion of cognition into her new social theory of emotion, which is explored further in Chapter 4.

Third, a significant aspect of patient vulnerability was clearly evident in Vignette 3. The patient is vulnerable because his physical illness was the reason for his need for medical care – and for emotional labour as part of that care. The prime emotion elicited due to the situation was anxiety which had a physical manifestation over which he had only a degree of control. His need was real, as was the potential for inflicting great pain during the removal of the drain. The emotional labour was seen to be essential in two respects. It was important in facilitating the patient's trust in his nurse based on her understanding of the situation. That understanding involved identifying the source and implication of his anxiety which was seen as being both biological and psychological. Thus, as the nurse, I held power over my patient in how I wielded that knowledge and executed the clinical task. For my emotional labour to be effective it was essential that I understood its physical manifestation in addition to the cognitive evaluations being shared in anticipation of the drain removal.

Fourth, in addition to the desire to care for my patient by managing his anxiety and minimising his pain and discomfort, the emotional labour in Vignette 3 was motivated in two further ways. The vignette begins by explaining that during this particular shift, I had time to carry out my duties more fully, an important point that is reiterated later when I note that 'what was so great about this was that I had time to do it properly'. The focus is on the task and the anticipation of performing it well. Carrying out effective emotional labour was an essential component to the degree of satisfaction I achieved as result of a job well done: this was a personal reward. However, in succeeding at the task I also received gratitude and approbation from the patients. I helped manage their anxieties, helping them to feel cared for; in turn, they rewarded me with gratitude. An emotion exchange took place, therefore, within the therapeutic relationship. Developing an understanding of the nature of emotion enables the identification and acknowledgement of the importance of these emotions to the value and need for emotional labour.

Hochschild's conceptualisation of the relationship between emotion and cognition is arguably limited because she does not engage with the organismic debate concerning the independence of emotion from cognition. She does, however, incorporate an understanding of the biological character of emotion. 'Since the body readies itself for action in physiological ways, emotion involves biological processes' (Hochschild 1983: 220). This chapter has explored Hochschild's conceptualisation of emotion and cognition which she examines at the beginning of Appendix A before she explores the organismic school. How she arrives at this conceptualisation, and the argument she develops to support it, subsequently becomes an underlying assumption that influences how she interprets Darwin and Freud and integrates them with interactionist approaches to emotion. This is examined in Chapter 4.

Vignette 4 'The murderer'

Catherine: Have you been in an emergency situation on the ward?

Susan: Yeah, I had a patient die on me. Didn't I tell you? I had the relatives telling me that I had murdered their sister!

No! Tell me about that.

She came up from A & E and she was struggling with her breathing and everything. She was under the urologists so I got the urology reg. [registrar] to come and see her, and I did everything right. And he said to me, 'Well she is totally stable', but I said, 'We can't get a blood pressure on her!', but they said, 'She's absolutely fine!' so I got the on call surgical SHO [senior house officer] to look at her as well, because I wasn't happy. And he said, 'Well, she is stable, don't worry, blah, blah, blah, but put up some gelofusin and get her blood pressure back up and everything'. And then I went on my break and I told Maxine [E grade nurse] everything. And then I got called back from my break because . . . When I left she was sitting up drinking, finding it hard to breathe, couldn't get a blood pressure, but she was a big lady anyway, so the dynomap [machine for taking blood pressure readings] wouldn't have worked, and I came back from my break and she was totally unresponsive. And we had to call the crash team and everything because we thought she was going to go. But they made her NFR [not for resuscitation] before that happened anyway. And then her sister rang up and she had been told while I was at break that she wasn't well and she called me a murderer because I told her that she had been put not for resus. And she said that I was murdering her sister and denying her the chance to live, which made me feel like a complete shit. God! They did apologise though, but it still didn't help. I went home. I was really gutted and I cried at home to Mum. It made me feel awful.

I remember that patient, I was on nights and I had to look after the relatives.

Yes, they arrived, and they did apologise the next day when they come up to get her stuff and everything. Still.

How did it make you feel when they said that to you on the phone?

I felt like a murderer. I felt guilty and it was horrible. It was just really you think to yourself, did I do enough? Did I get the right people to see her? Did I do everything? If I had done all of this would she be all right now? But at the end of the day she was riddled with cancer and resuscitating her would have been, well, it would have been horrible for her. Let her die with some dignity you know. And I felt bad for Maxine because although I had explained everything, I'd gone off and she was sitting up, drinking and talking and I'd come back and she was flat on her back and unresponsive, you know, it's just like, what the hell happened? And at the end, Ann [student nurse] said, 'Don't worry about it, forget it' and I was thinking, 'You haven't got a clue, you can forget it 'cos you are the student, but I am responsible for her [the patient] and it's just . . . And although it wasn't actually an arrest everything was done as if it had've been, all apart from resuscitating.'

Did you feel like kicking it all in?

No. It made me more determined, to remember for next time to do things a bit differently.

How would you have dealt with it differently?

When she first came up on the ward, because A & E had told me that they had phoned the relatives in the morning, and when she came up on the ward, she was quite ill, so I think I would have phoned the relatives then. Then they would have been there by the time all of that had happened. That is the first thing I would have done differently. But then you don't, you see, I mean how many situations do you look back, how many situations has that happened and you don't, and people die and then you ring the relatives and it is too late. And I was praying, you know, because they got there before she died didn't they? And I was going, '*Please* hold on for your sister' and I was really begging her!

Yeah, I put her into a side room, to give them some space.

Mm, I really was begging her to hold on because I knew that once her sister got there and saw what a state she was in, she would agree to the NFR status, but if she had died before she got there she would never have known what she had been like and she would still think that we had been, that we had just said it willy-nilly, wouldn't she? Oh, it was horrible.

I don't think the sister knew that she had got cancer.

No, she didn't.

So it was a shock. I remember that.

But they did apologise, but even so.

Did it make you feel physically sick?

Yes it did. I think it was the adrenaline, I think that the adrenaline makes you sick doesn't it? Terrible!

4 Synthesising Darwin and Freud with interactionist theory

Hochschild's approach to cognition is ultimately one which supports her prioritisation of social factors in her new theory of emotion. This is unsurprising, as Hochschild does develop a *social* theory. However, it also suggests that her theory is not as inclusive of biopsycho approaches as others have claimed (S. Williams 1998a). Chapter 4 demonstrates this by looking at *how* she integrates Darwin's theory of gesture and Freud's notion of the conscious and unconscious mind, with social interactionists Dewey, Gerth and Mills, Mead and Goffman. Identifying the significance of this prioritisation in the formulation of her theory is important, because it underpins how she conceptualises emotion management, surface and deep acting and the self. Restricting the relevance of the biopsycho nature of emotion results in these concepts having significant limitations, which impacts on how the process of emotion management is understood to occur, and in how it is related to the self. This is significant to nursing, because it is Hochschild's notion of emotion management that has been applied to it.

Synthesising Darwin and Freud

Darwin's (1872) focus in his book *The Expression of the Emotions in Man and Animals* is on the outward, visible gestures that convey emotional expression from one person to another, such as smiling or grimacing. He argues that such expressions are directly related to primitive man. Love derives from the act of copulation, the expression of disgust from regurgitation and so on. Hochschild accepts that gesture is part of the physical manifestation of emotion but does not comment on Darwin's analysis of the origin of emotion which supports Zajonc's (1984) assertion that emotion biologically precedes cognition on the evolutionary scale. Instead she engages with the cultural debate on whether physical gestures communicating emotion are universal and innate, or culturally variable. Is it the case that when an American person smiles it means the same as an Aborigine, African or Inuit? Hochschild argues that the debate itself is inadequate because it misses out 'a conception of emotion as [a] subjective experience and a more subtle and complex notion of how social factors impinge' (1983: 208).

She implies that as a subjective experience, emotion is culturally variable. This is the extent of her use of Darwin, resulting in the physical experience of emotion being reduced to one of gesture. Next, Hochschild shows how she moves from physical gesture as an orientation towards action to emotion an orientation towards cognition. To do this she draws from Freud's analysis of anxiety to link the two through the relationship of the conscious and unconscious mind.

Freud suggests that the unconscious mind acts as a mediator between an instinctive reaction (such as fear represented by the id) and individual understanding of social influences (the degree of the threat – represented by the ego). Emotions therefore, are seen as signals that precipitate action. Freud claims that it is the role of the ego 'to postpone id drives, to neutralise them or bind them' (Hochschild 1983: 208–209). In order for the mind to make this distinction, the meaning of the emotion is essential. However, Hochschild notes that for Freud the meaning may be unconscious. She quotes Freud:

> To begin with it may happen that an affect or an emotion is perceived, but misconstrued. By the repression of its proper presentation it is forced to become connected with another idea, and is now interpreted by consciousness as this expression of this other idea. If we restore the true connection, we call the original affect 'unconscious' although the affect was never unconscious but its ideational presentation had undergone repression.
>
> (Freud 1915a: 110, cited in Hochschild 1983: 210)

For example if we imagine a nurse reacting to a patient who vomits, what Freud suggests is that the nurse actually feels disgust towards the patient, but represses the feeling. In doing so, the nurse's conscious mind interprets her feeling as empathy, and her actions as caring and kindness. The feeling of disgust is not actually unconscious; it is repressed by the ideational presentation of the nurse as kind. Freud's conceptualisation of the relationship between the id and the ego allows for cognitive emotion management by giving the ego the role of the mediator, interpreting the unconscious mind and repressing certain emotions which the id is seeking to express.

Hochschild then briefly mentions other biological approaches towards emotion, commenting on the work of William James (1884) as equating 'emotion with bodily change and visceral feeling' (Hochschild 1983: 211). She acknowledges the debate over the relationship between physiological expression of emotion and cognitive appraisal, but dismisses it as inadequate in accounting for human emotion. Instead she suggests that what needs to be examined is 'how cultural rules might (through the superego) apply to the ego's operations (emotion work) on id (feeling)' (Hochschild 1983: 210). To do this, Hochschild turns to the interactionist school.

Synthesising Dewey and Gerth and Mills with Mead and Goffman

Hochschild's introduction to the interactionist school clearly states her reading of its relationship with the organismic school:

> The organismic view reduces us to an elicitation-expression model. The interactional model presupposes biology but adds more points to social entry: social factors enter not simply before and after but interactively *during* the experience of emotion . . . *By virtue of its greater complexity, the interactional model poses a choice between models of how social factors work.*
>
> (Hochschild 1983: 211–212, original emphasis)

Here Hochschild clearly reduces organismic understandings of emotion to one of elicitation-expression, and increases the significance of social factors. To illustrate this, she systematically highlights aspects of Dewey, Gerth and Mills, Mead and Goffman's work. She then synthesises them to build an integrated approach to emotion, revisiting how her interactionist approach works with the organismic approach outlined above.

Dewey and Gerth and Mills suggest that interaction shapes and defines emotion experiences, in that 'each feeling takes its shape and in a sense only becomes itself in social context' (Hochschild 1983: 212). Like Darwin, their focus is on gesture, not as universal and innate signals, but as signals which can be interpreted in response to a social situation or a social structure/ institution. For example, Gerth and Mills (1964) argue, if a bride has been jilted at the altar and cries, and the mother defines the crying as a sign of anger, then the bride will interpret the emotion as anger. Other people therefore, can influence an individual's understanding of their feelings, and even change them. Hochschild links this approach to Mead's (1934) idea of the self. He differentiated between the 'spontaneous uncontrolled "I"' and the reflective, directing, monitoring "Me"' (Hochschild 1983: 212). Hochschild claims that if Mead had developed a theory of emotion he may have introduced differences within the 'I' based on interaction. Together, Hochschild uses these theorists to demonstrate how interaction can shape, define and even change people's emotions. This is a valuable approach which illustrates the importance of emotion to social interaction and vice versa.

Hochschild then develops two of Goffman's ideas. Goffman identified the importance of understanding that successful social interaction takes constant 'work'. The need for *work* suggests there is the potential to not conform, but to express whatever one feels like. Thus, Hochschild (1983: 214) argues: 'the individual's social feelings are not repressed and made unconscious as they are for Freud but consciously suppressed or controlled'. Goffman also looks at what motivates people to conform. He suggests that conformity results in membership of the social community. Emotions, such as embarrassment and fear, indicate that individuals care what the community thinks of them. Conformity is encouraged through rules which 'establish a sense of obligation and license as they apply to the microacts of seeing, thinking about, remembering, recognising, feeling, or displaying' (Hochschild 1983: 215). When a person gets the rules wrong, acting in socially unacceptable ways, they experience embarrassment and shame. Goffman links the self with rules and emotion, based on social factors. Thus, through Goffman, Hochschild integrates emotion within sociological concepts concerning social regulation and integration, rules, values and norms. However, Hochschild also criticises his approach:

> Goffman shows us the self coming alive only in a social situation where display to other people is an issue. We are invited to ignore all moments in which the individual introspects or dwells on outer reality without a sense of watchers. Thus, guilt, the sign of a broken *internalized* rule, is seldom, if ever discussed. To discuss it would be to put the rule 'inside' the actor, inside a sort of self that Goffman does not deal with.
> (Hochschild 1983: 216, original emphasis)

Hochschild suggests that Goffman's self is a surface one with a lack of depth and a lack of ownership of its own emotion experiences and responses. 'Goffman speaks as if his actors can induce or prevent, or suppress feeling – as if they had the capacity to shape emotion. But what is the relation between this *capacity to act* and the self?' (Hochschild 1983: 217, original emphasis). To answer this, Hochschild turns back to Freud's notion of the id, the ego and the superego, which negotiates conscious and unconscious emotion and shows a self 'that could feel and manage feeling' (1983: 217).

Hochschild's new social theory of emotion

Drawing them together, Hochschild (1983: 219) synthesises these organismic and interactionist approaches into her new social theory of emotion as a sense that is 'related not only to an orientation towards action but also towards cognition':

> Emotion is our experience of the body ready for imaginary action. Since the body readies itself for action in physiological ways, emotion involves biological processes. Thus when we manage an emotion we are partly managing a bodily preparation for a consciously or unconsciously anticipated deed. This is why emotion work is work . . . Cognition is involved in the process by which emotions 'signal' messages to the individual . . . But signalling is complex . . . it involves a reality newly grasped on the template of prior expectations . . . The idea of prior expectations implies the existence of a prior self . . . Most of us maintain a prior expectation of a continuous self, but the character of self we

expect to maintain is subject to profoundly social influence. In so far as our self and all we expect is social – the way emotion signals messages to us is also influenced by social factors.

(Hochschild 1983: 220–222)

Hochschild acknowledges the centrality of the physiological experience and process of emotion, including it in her definition of emotion management. She identifies that the elicitation of physiological emotion occurs in response to conscious and unconscious anticipation. This anticipation is based on previous and remembered experiences, central to the idea and development of 'self' and is inherently social. Hochschild links, therefore, how emotion signals messages to us through anticipated remembered, conscious and unconscious processes, built on the template of prior expectations formulated by social factors (Theodosius 2006).

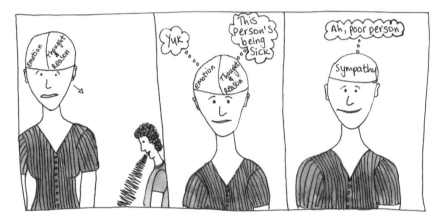

'Emotion work'

**Hochschild's new social theory of emotion in 'The murderer'
(Vignette 4)**

'Emotion is the experience of the body ready for imaginary action': Susan describes how her patient was admitted to the ward from A & E requiring emergency treatment. Susan's body, in the release of emotion, physiologically readied itself, enabling her to work towards stabilising her patient's condition. The emotion is strong enough to motivate her to seek a second opinion from a doctor whom she knows better, when she is unhappy over the urology registrar's actions. The emotion elicited is connected to her conscious cognitive anticipation that her patient is likely to crash. Susan interprets the emotion as being anxiety because she is anxious to ensure that she gives her the best possible care if this should occur. This conscious understanding is based on her pre-existing knowledge about the physiological symptoms of the body which she anticipates might result in cardiac arrest, so she works to stabilise it. Thus, Susan's anxiety about her patient's well-being precipitates her actions on her behalf.

However, a decision is made by the medical team not to resuscitate this patient in the event of a cardiac arrest, as it is deemed inappropriate. Having been informed of this when the sister calls, she accuses Susan of being a murderer. This social interaction causes Susan to consciously reinterpret her emotion as guilt based on internalised feeling rules that suggest she is responsible for her patient's health, wellbeing and safety. She now feels that she has not done enough and questions the care she has given: 'for even though it wasn't an arrest everything was done as if it had've been'.

However, through continuing cognitive process, Susan consciously works on the feeling of guilt, acknowledging that to resuscitate the patient would be cruel. Thus, she attempts to induce the emotion of sympathy. She does this by acknowledging that death will be a blessing for her patient, who is riddled with cancer. This elicits sympathy, which she can now extend to the sister, who will be bereaved. Her emotion work includes her begging the patient not to die before her sister arrives, so that she can realise this for herself. Through her emotion work, Susan acts out the feeling rule in which the nurse facilitates a dignified and peaceful death in the case of the patient, and feels sympathy for the grieving relatives.

Hochschild's new social theory of emotion develops a biopsychosocial approach, linked to the self and based on social interaction. However, the centrality of emotion, its interactive nature and its connection to the self, is lost when Hochschild applies it to surface acting and deep acting, feeling rules and emotion management. This is because difficulties in her interpretation and the integration of the different theorists, becomes more relevant at this point.

As noted in Chapter 1, Hochschild directly links surface and deep acting with Stanislavski's method acting, and Goffman's notion of dramaturgy.

> We all do a certain amount of acting. But we may act in two different ways. In the first way, we try to change how we outwardly appear. As it is for the people observed by Erving Goffman, the action is in the body language, the put on sneer, the posed shrug, the controlled sigh. This is

surface acting. The other way is deep acting. Here display is a natural result of working on feeling; the actor does not try to seem happy or sad but rather expresses spontaneously . . . a real feeling that has been self induced.

(Hochschild 1983: 35)

It is possible to see here how Hochschild synthesises the biological, psychological and the social in her notion of surface and deep acting. In surface acting she brings together Darwin's theory of gesture and Goffman's individual acting for social effect. In deep acting she brings together Goffman's notion of the individual *working* to create the right effect and Freud's more complex ego mediator role between the real self (id) and the social self (superego). In surface acting Hochschild overcomes her difficulty with Darwin by making social factors essential to interpreting gesture. In deep acting she develops Goffman's surface self by showing how the self has the ability to internalise social rules in her use of Freud. In surface acting, the actor knows what gestures to act out according to feeling rules, social norms and values. In deep acting, the actor internalises these rules. Her integration of these different theories in her development of surface and deep acting and her notion of feeling rules is fundamental. However, in the synthesis of these different approaches, Hochschild integrates the social with the physiological and the social with the psychological. She does not integrate all three together, thereby creating a true biopsychosocial approach. This is because in the creation of a social theory of emotion, she fundamentally develops a social interactionist approach to emotion, in which social factors are primary.

For the interactionist it is highly questionable that feeling is present all along. How do we know, they ask, that the very focusing of attention and use of cognitive power does not in itself evoke the feeling? And if the act of attending to feeling shapes the feeling itself, that feeling cannot be referred to independently of these acts. Similarly, the act of management is inseparable from the experience that is managed; it is in part the *creation* of that emerging experience. Just as knowing affects what is known, so managing affects what is 'there' to be managed . . . [Thus], in the interactionist model, social factors enter *into the very formulation* of emotions, through codification, management and expression.

(Hochschild 1983: 206–207, original emphasis)

However, bringing 'social factors into the very formulation of emotion' generates significant theoretical difficulties. This is because interaction actually takes place between the creation and management of emotion, and feeling rules. The importance of social interaction between people in the creation and interpretation of emotion becomes less significant. In the process, emotion also becomes subject to cognition, and always being inherently manageable reduces emotion to ideas that 'have no autonomy from the rational world with which they coexist' (Craib 1995: 153). Thus, the value of using Darwin and Freud in representing the biopsycho aspects of emotion in her theory is reduced, because the idea that emotion does not always lend itself to being managed and can sometimes be unconscious, is lost. Together, these difficulties also impact on her notion of the 'self' because ultimately the self interacts with fixed – almost reified – feeling rules that have become objectified whether they are external or internalised. Thus, Hochschild's notion of emotion management/labour as something that 'requires one to induce or suppress feelings in order to sustain the outward countenance that produces the proper state of mind in others' (1983: 7) assumes that, first, it is always possible to manage one's emotions, second, that this can be achieved through the work of the emotional labourer alone, and third, the interaction between the emotional labourer and the recipient is one way because the interaction is really with feeling rules. Equally, while 'this kind of labour calls for the coordination of mind and feeling, and it sometimes draws on a source of self that we honour as deep and integral to our individuality' (Hochschild 1983: 7), it is acted out using processes of deception in either surface or deep acting. The degree of deception is based on object-like feeling rules that are either surface or internalised. Thus Hochschild's self is either deceived or deceiving. Her focus on social factors and the belief that emotion always lends itself to being managed also limits her notions of surface and deep acting because they represent the process of emotion management and are integral to the self.

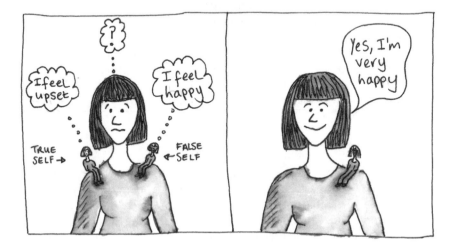

'Self-deception'

---

*Inauthenticity and self-deception in the application of
Hochschild's new social theory of emotion in 'The murderer'
(Vignette 4)*

In the initial analysis of the vignette, Susan's emotions were identified by associating them with feeling rules. The role of the interactions that took place between various people became less relevant, even though the interaction between Susan and the sister which took place over the phone was initially considered.

Equally, Susan's emotion management in which she expresses sympathy to the sister involves deception. Either she is deceiving herself or the sister, in order to carry out her emotional labour. We know this because Susan not only cries when she gets home, but also states that the sister's apology was not enough.

Ultimately, using Hochschild's approach, Susan's sympathy is inauthentic and she has deceived either herself or the sister, which results in a degree of self-alienation from her own emotions.

Equally, following through the previous analysis, it would seem that Susan has successfully managed her emotion. However, the narrative was first introduced when Susan was asked if she had ever been in an emergency situation before. Her reply to that was 'Yeah, I had a patient die on me. Didn't I tell you? I had the relatives telling me that I had murdered their sister!' This statement implies responsibility – the patient died on me. The following statement – when the relatives accused her of being a murderer – implies the awfulness of that responsibility to Susan. The emotions of guilt and horror at what happened are still very strong some months after the event, even though both statements are inaccurate. The patient actually died during the night on my shift, and Susan certainly did not murder her. The exaggeration in these statements enables Susan to communicate the strength of her feelings of shock, horror and guilt. This suggests that perhaps Susan has not really managed her emotions at all.

Surface acting

These limitations are clearly evident in her notion of surface acting. For example, the surface actor knowingly sets out to portray socially expected emotions that they do not really feel, in order to deceive others. Often, the deception does indeed pass undetected. However, sometimes the audience may realise that they are not seeing 'real' or sincere feelings, but due to social norms, accept the performance at face value. For example, when introduced at a social gathering, an individual may smile and affect pleasure in meeting others, even though they will probably instantaneously forget their name and be unlikely to meet them again. The social rules governing this exchange, however, are important: although no one is deceived by the projected sentiments they would be insulted if the formalities were not followed (Goffman 1959, 1961, 1967). Hochschild does not include this double 'deception', because she examines only the emotional labourer's perspective, and that perspective is solely informed by feeling rules. It is also possible that while the actor may intend to deceive others about their real feelings, they may not be successful. This could be because their body language unintentionally gives them away when their emotions are difficult to manage (Duck 1998; Layder 2004a, 2004b). Or, it might be because those with whom they are interacting *know* them, and are well aware what their probable emotions really are. This is where interaction *between* people, and *who* those people are, is as pertinent to understanding the emotions being expressed and managed, as the social context is.

Hochschild (1990) develops her idea of surface acting further in 'Ideology and emotion management', suggesting that it is possible to 'change feeling from the "outside in"'. Here surface acting becomes similar to deep acting because by changing outward expression it is possible to intentionally change inward feeling too. She gives the example of a flight attendant who says, 'If I pretend I'm feeling really up, sometimes I actually cheer up and feel friendly. The passenger responds to me as though I were friendly and then more of me responds back' (Hochschild 1990: 121). Here the surface acting becomes more real because of the response of the *other* person. By introducing an interactive element to surface acting, Hochschild almost changes the definition, in that it becomes part of the process in working towards deep acting, as the flight attendant actually cheers up and believes that she is friendly. In fact in her notes at the end of *The Managed Heart*, Hochschild does define this kind of acting as deep acting using a surface-centred approach.

> Th[e] surface-to-centre approach differs from surface acting. Surface acting uses the body to *show* feeling. This type of deep acting uses the body to *inspire* feeling. In relaxing a grimace or unclenching a fist, we may actually make ourselves feel less angry.
> (Hochschild 1983: 247, original emphasis)

The definition here is specific to deep acting, but in 'Ideology and emotion management' (1990) she equates it with surface acting. It becomes like deep acting because she introduces a motivational and interactional aspect to the process. It is also possible that when interaction occurs, emotions are generated between people, transcending each individual. It is equally possible that the nature of emotion management is different when both people are managing or expressing emotion within a dynamic interactive encounter. Hochschild's notion of surface acting therefore can be developed further by introducing a more interactive element.

Surface acting in 'The murderer' (Vignette 4)

Susan uses surface acting in the management of her anxiety and guilt. Her anxiety is surface deep because it motivates her actions: she notes at the end of the passage that the adrenaline made her feel sick. She uses the anxiety to precipitate her actions, sufficiently suppressing it so that it does not control her. During the telephone conversation with the patient's sister, Susan also surface acts. However, the sister is not deceived about how Susan feels, despite her acting. This is evident when she apologises to her. Susan uses surface acting when she accepts the apology as well, commenting that it did not help. It is possible that Susan finds the apology inadequate because the sister is also using surface acting when making it. After all, she is in a state of shock and grief. There is a sense that *each* person is acting out social forms here. Susan uses surface acting in her role as the nurse who understands and cares about how the sister is feeling. The sister uses surface acting when she apologises, in her role as the recipient of care. The apology is an acknowledgement of that care. Both trust the other to perform according to the social norms and feeling rules. Neither participant however, is actually deceived. Each knows that what has occurred is awful and neither feel exonerated about their role in it.

Social factors that include interaction between people in the expression and management of emotion are important in understanding the nature of Susan's emotion management. However, they do not fully explain it. Despite the social interaction which should either expiate the guilt, or result in its reinterpretation, Susan still feels guilty.

Deep acting

In deep acting, Hochschild focuses on how feeling rules are internalised, changing feelings 'from the "inside out"' (1990: 120). As noted in Chapter 1, this can be done by exhorting emotion, using imagination and through emotion memory. Hochschild's synthesis of Freud with interactionism is more successful here. The motivation for deep acting can come from external social factors, such as feeling rules, but its process is an internal one, a relationship between mind and body and within the mind itself. Use of imagination or emotion memory as a means of stimulating emotion is important in two ways. First, it suggests a degree of anticipation, bringing the self from the present and taking it through to the future based on past experience. This is what Hochschild (1990: 220) means when she talks about emotions signalling through cognition messages based on prior experience that are integrally representative of the self. This process can be both conscious and unconscious. In this way emotion becomes a means of motivating action. Second, it develops the idea that the mind can use the body to release emotion which it anticipates feeling, and in the release of that emotion come to actually experience it. This is seen in the example of the flight attendant who aspired to feel cheerful. This process is important in understanding the embodiment of emotion and the relationship between mind, body and society (Freund 1990; Archer 2000). However, despite Hochschild's inclusion of unconscious process, the process she describes is largely conscious.

For example, although Hochschild writes about emotion memory as if it can be unconscious, she does so from the perspective of it being formulated, managed and expressed through external social factors based on conscious cognitive processes. Thus deep acting is seen as being based on processes of deception. Hochschild suggests that through emotion memory and imagi-nation, emotion can be created. In this way emotion responses are learned. The link between that learning and social factors, such as feeling rules, does not necessarily mean that individuals have deceived themselves about the authenticity of the emotions they subsequently experience. If this was the case all forms of learning would be based on patterns of self-deception. Although Hochschild includes unconscious emotion within her theory, she talks about deep acting as involving 'work' in the production of more socially acceptable emotion expression, which is a conscious process. While it *is* possible to consciously draw on emotion memory, it is *also* possible to act by rote due to previous learned behaviours or habit. Bourdieu (1990) would suggest that such behaviour is pre-reflexive, in that it is habitual, and does not require reflexive or conscious thought. In this way, emotion behaviour can be learnt using conscious processes; then it becomes pre-reflexive seeping into habitual behaviour. If this is the case, it suggests that such emotions are

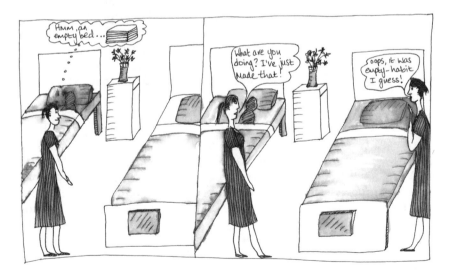

'Empty bed syndrome'

embodied, and integral to self-identity, forming pre-reflexive emotion expressions and responses that are indicative of individual character. Pre-reflexive action is neither conscious nor unconscious. Pre-reflexive action based on habit is more representative of what Hochschild is striving to suggest than the idea that unconscious emotion, which influences deep acting, is based on deception. The idea of a pre-reflexive emotion memory which is individual to the self therefore, impacts on how the self anticipates in the present, and projects into the future based on past experiences of the prior self. An understanding of how this is achieved and its connection to processes of emotion management is required to develop Hochschild's notion of deep acting.

Emotion memory

In addition to being pre-reflexive, cognitive processes can be unconscious and can also influence emotion memory (LeDoux 1998; Kihlstrom et al. 2000; Strongman 2003). Equally, emotion memory can be unconscious and bypass cognitive processes altogether, thereby influencing actions in ways that are not manageable (LeDoux 1998). Both neuroscientists and cognitive psychologists agree that memory can be both conscious and unconscious, the difference between them being defined as 'explicit' and 'implicit' memory (Schacter 1987; LeDoux 1998; Kihlstrom et al. 2000; Strongman 2003). Explicit memory refers to conscious awareness in social action, whereas implicit memory refers to the guiding of action by unconscious factors (LeDoux 1998; Kihlstrom et al. 2000; Strongman 2003). Emotion, however, is central to conscious explicit memory because it makes it more real (LeDoux 1998). This is because neural stimulation of conscious memory and emotional arousal within the hippocampus and neocortex (conscious memory), and stimulation in the amygdala (emotion arousal) occurs together. However, 'sensual stimuli can trigger an [implicit] emotion memory *without* triggering explicit cognitive memory. This experience of being emotionally aroused and not knowing why is all too common to us' (LeDoux 1998: 203, my emphasis). Thus emotion memory can be unconscious, stimulated by touch, taste, sight, sound and smell, triggers that are *sensual*. These triggers reflect the embodied presence of individuals within the entire environment and not just the social context. Thus the body can act before it is aware of what it is reacting too. How emotion is elicited in response to interaction with the natural and material world is something Hochschild does not include in her new social theory of emotion.

These experiences are stored in the implicit emotion memory, and are unconscious. However, while the function of emotion within the brain is part of unconscious processes, *conscious* emotional feeling is impossible without emotional experience also being represented in the explicit, working memory (LeDoux 1998). 'Working memory is the gateway to subjective experiences, emotional and non-emotional ones, and is indispensible in the creation of conscious emotion feeling' (LeDoux 1998: 296). In this respect, when Hochschild (1983) notes that consciously exhorting or imagining emotion can actually make people feel the way they want to by working on their emotions, this involves their *explicit working* memory. Thus her notion of emotion memory is tenable; however, it is not the whole picture because individuals also have an unconscious implicit emotion memory that can supersede conscious processes:

> Contrary to the primary supposition of cognitive appraisal theories, the core of an emotion is not an introspectively accessible conscious representation. Feelings do involve conscious content, but we don't necessarily have conscious access to the processes that produce the content. And even when we do have introspective access, the conscious content is not likely to be what triggered the emotional responses in the first place. The emotional responses and the conscious content are both products of specialised emotion systems that operate unconsciously.
>
> (LeDoux 1998: 299)

Hochschild's notion of emotion as being like a sense has resonance here; however LeDoux's representation develops its orientation towards action and identifies the mechanism involved in its orientation towards cognition further. For, its orientation towards action is linked to both implicit and explicit emotion memory in a way that both bypasses and connects with cognition. This representation has implications in how emotion is connected with self-identity. For Hochschild, the connection to the self comes with her use of Freud in the internalisation of social factors.

Deep acting and emotion memory in 'The murderer' (Vignette 4)

Deep acting involves the internalisation of feeling rules based on a relationship between the mind and the body, and within the mind itself. Hochschild integrates the self – in the form of the past self – as aiding cognitive understanding of the import of the situation either through emotion memory or through imagination.

There is evidence in the vignette that Susan is acting on internalised feeling rules and social norms. It is her responsibility to care for the patient and ensure her safety and wellbeing. She comments: 'I am responsible for her and it's just . . . And although it wasn't actually an arrest everything was done as if it had've been, all apart from resuscitating.' Susan does not appear to be entirely convinced by her own rationale. This is the *first* experience Susan has had of an emergency situation. Her difficulty with the internalised feeling rule, therefore, is that the emergency situation is not associated with past emotions; she has no emotion memory. The opening question, initiating this account, is about this. Susan is a newly qualified staff nurse in her first post (she was the student nurse in Vignette 3). Training for cardio-pulmonary-resuscitation (CPR) is rigorous and extensive. The idea is to be able to act almost without thought in order to override panic, and so that each individual always knows how to act in that situation. Susan's pre-reflexive response is ready. However, emotionally she has not experienced this before. This pre-reflexive knowledge is not associated with feelings based on past experience. Therefore, Susan is still trying to make sense of how she feels about what has happened. She uses the internalised feeling rule about responsibility and duty of care to help her, but she is not sure whether it is appropriate because it is somewhat disconnected from the resuscitation process, which didn't really happen despite the fact that she did actually do everything correctly.

The duty of care she has towards her patient dominates her thinking. She applies it to Maxine trying to justify going on her break, and she is angry when the student does not understand it. It also gives credence to her self-doubt and feelings of guilt.

Thus, the anxiety that Susan felt in the outset becomes confused by the patient's sister's angry accusation that she is guilty of not caring for her patient properly. Susan's subsequent behaviour and actions suggest that she believes that she is guilty. For example, she tries to use her imagination to induce sympathy for the sister, but she does so because she wants to persuade the sister that she is not really guilty. At the end of the vignette, when asked what she would do differently, it is interesting that she would inform the sister about her patient's condition earlier. This is a recognition that for the patient, she did everything as well as she could under the circumstances. But it is also an acknowledgement of guilt towards the sister. The guilt is connected with the sister not the patient – but the justification is connected to feeling rules associated with her responsibility for her patient's safety. The guilt and the anxiety are interconnected, impacting on each other.

Thus, throughout the vignette, it seems that Susan is giving a rational explanation in which she knows that she is not guilty, she did every-thing right. Despite this, the emotions associated with it are ones of guilt and horror at the awfulness. These are the emotions that she remembers and which colour and make real that experience to her as she narrates it in the interview. These are arguably unconscious emotions, which through her implicit memory are associated with the events, despite her conscious repudiation of them. It is possible –

although unknown here – that future emergency situations may be coloured by unconscious feelings of guilt as well as anxiety.

There is also evidence that Susan feels quite angry about the situation. She is certainly indignant at the sister's accusation. She appears to be struggling with feeling angry about the whole situation but cannot really justify or verbalise why. This may be because guilt is still impeding her from accepting the sister's unjustified accusation, despite her cognitive acknowledgement of it and has become associated with the feeling of anxiety elicited at the onset of the situation and linked to her belief that it was her responsibility to save the sister.

Hochschild's notion of deep acting is useful; however, it is also simplistic. Susan is attempting to manage at least three emotions here, each connected to similar feeling rules. How they are connected to her sense of self-identity however, is not clear.

Freud and the unconscious

'Through Freud, I circle back from the organismic to the interactional tradition, tracing through an analysis of the signal function of feeling how social factors influence what we expect and thus what feelings "signal"' (Hochschild 1983: 222). Hochschild shows how social rules apply to what the individual thinks and displays using deep acting. In integrating interactionist theory with Freud, she builds on Mead's 'I', representing the spontaneous self, and his 'me' – the self that socially interacts (Hochschild 1983: 212). She does this by looking at the interface between the 'I' and the 'me' to explain how an individual manages conflicting social rules and obligations that induce conformity of action and yet can chose to deviate from them (Goffman 1967, 1969). She suggests that 'spontaneous emotion', until it has become socially interactive, is not necessarily identified in its moment of experience. Its interpretation is based on cultural difference. Thus, through the impact of social interactionism on the 'I' Hochschild renders the self subject of its emotion in its capacity to act, that is the individual can now feel and manage emotion. Using this, she reinterprets Freud, bringing his notion of emotion repression into an interactionist framework, suggesting 'that the individual's social feelings are not repressed and made unconscious, as they are for Freud, but consciously suppressed or controlled' (Hochschild 1983: 214).

Hochschild runs into some difficulties here. First, as she notes, Freud actually argues that an individual's feelings are not really unconscious but repressed. Second rather than talking about 'original feelings' being *repressed*, Hochschild is now talking about 'social feelings' being *suppressed*. This is because in Freud, the original emotion is part of the role of the id, being spontaneous and instinctive. The 'I' in Mead is represented as spontaneous and not socially different and is similar therefore, to Freud's id, but Hochschild has reinterpreted Mead's 'I' as being culturally variable and socially different, which makes it too similar to the 'me' and to Freud's superego. What she gains in using Freud and Mead to bring a more detailed and developed understanding of psychology to the individual therefore, she loses because she links emotion to consciously managed social factors. Thus, within her theory, there is no room for 'original' emotions, only socially managed ones. This creates a dichotomy between 'real', 'authentic' feelings and 'managed', 'social' feelings, and Hochschild's self then mimics this division, dividing into the 'true' self and the 'false' self as a result of emotion management.

A further difference between Hochschild and Freud is that for Freud, the original emotion *appears* unconscious only because of its conscious ideational presentation resulting in its repression. Because it is repressed, rather than unconscious, it is somewhat volatile, allowing for the possibility that emotion is not always manageable. For Freud notes, the original emotion is conscious, but it is unacknowledged because it has been misconstrued by the conscious through the process of ideational presentation which has repressed it. The conscious mind erroneously thinks that it is now unconscious. Consequently, the emotion has not really been managed, making it unpredictable and volatile. As repressed emotion is by nature unacknowledged, it may express, influence or motivate further emotion responses, and bypass cognitive processes. Freud's approach to reason (associated with social factors) suggests that what is unconscious must first emerge into preconscious perception becoming associated with ideas in order to become conscious; however, feelings can override this process. Thus, conscious and unconscious emotion, which directly impact on both internal and external behaviour patterns, can bypass cognitive processes:

> With unconscious ideas connecting links must be created before they can be brought into the conscious, with feelings . . . , this does not occur. In other words, the distinction between the conscious and preconscious has no meaning where feelings are concerned . . . ; feelings are either conscious or unconscious. Even when they are attached to word-presentations, their becoming conscious is not due to that circumstance, but they become so directly.
>
> (Freud 2001 [1923]: 22–23)

Using Freud's definition of repression, and conscious and unconscious feelings, there is scope for emotion to override cognitive control imposed by the superego because both conscious and unconscious emotion can emerge directly without being associated with word-presentations representing social factors. That conscious, cognitive management of emotion renders it open to processes of reason is clearly possible: emotion, however, can also precipitate irrational action, which resists attempts to override, control or

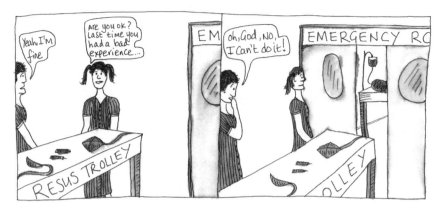

'Sudden panic'

manage it. Freud's theory here is similar to current neuroscientific understandings of the relationship between cognition and emotion represented
in the difference between implicit and explicit memory (LeDoux 1998).
In fact within Freud's analysis, it is also possible that conscious emotion
management – which represses an emotion in order to express another one
in its place – may take place in order to facilitate other unconscious emotion
expressions. For example, the nurse who represses disgust and expresses
sympathy through the ideational presentation of herself as caring may be
fulfilling other unconscious emotion drives. For in the expression of sympathy she gives care and love, but she also receives love and gratitude in
return. There may be a deep unconscious need in her to be loved, which is
gratified by being needed by others. In this respect, the hidden emotion of
love is unconsciously motivating both the emotion management of the
disgust, and her social choice to do nursing.

This reading of Freud has four benefits. First, it accounts for the interactive
relationship between the id, ego and superego in a more balanced way. It
takes away the need to see deep acting as involving deception. Second,
allowing for unconscious emotion that can be *independent* of cognition and
unmanageable because it supersedes cognition or is unacknowledged, enables
a more balanced flow within the id–ego–superego self. This accounts for the
possibility that the self may experience conflicting emotions without breaking
down. This overcomes Hochschild's dualistic conflict between the 'real' and
'false' self, in which unconscious emotions not linked to social factors are
considered authentic and representative of the 'real' self. Third, it accounts
for emotions that are generated between people and the emotion exchanges
that take place. Such emotions are relevant to people's underlying needs that
are reflected within their characters and how they manage them within the
id–ego–superego relationship and consequently how they motivate their
actions. Fourth, it demonstrates how emotion expression and management

is not one-dimensional. Many emotions and feelings may be involved, being experienced, expressed and managed together.

Freud and the unconscious in 'The murderer' (Vignette 4)

The emotions of anxiety and guilt are clearly manifested throughout this vignette. There is also an undercurrent of anger and bewilderment. Susan has had to manage her first emergency experience. She has done everything in her power to care for this patient, including bringing in an additional doctor. Yet, the sister feels that it is acceptable to accuse Susan of murdering her sister. In fact, in the accusation, the sister is expressing *her* anger at the situation. This brings the emotion of anger into the interaction between them. Susan does not retaliate and become angry in return, instead she seems to embrace the implied guilt. It is possible that the ideational presentation of her role as a responsible nurse, an internalised feeling rule, acted upon in her concern and anticipation of the patient's imminent cardiac arrest, has resulted in her conscious mind interpreting her emotion as guilt. The emotion is not guilt, it is anger, but she believes that it is guilt despite her attempt to justify her actions and accept that she is not guilty. She is not able to do this, because the real emotion is not guilt but anger, which she does not acknowledge because it is repressed. It is possible that the anger is repressed because to acknowledge it would result in Susan admitting she is angry about someone who is grieving. This would be an act of unkindness and suggest that she is not a kind, caring nurse – feelings she has worked hard to induce. As a nurse, for whom caring and empathy is essential to her identity, this may be difficult to accept. This does not make her guilt less real or authentic. In fact it is arguable that she really feels guilty about her repressed anger towards the patient's sister. Thus, she cannot accept the sister's apology. Susan holds these different emotions in balance however, and uses them to motivate her to learn and respond differently in subsequent similar situations – thus maintaining her identity as a responsible, kind and caring nurse.

Conclusion

Hochschild's development of a biopsychosocial approach in her new social theory of emotion is unique. Integrating these different perspectives on emotion, however, is not without difficulty and the subsequent problems which arise from this are reflected in her notion of surface and deep acting, feeling rules and emotion management. Essentially she integrates bio-psycho perspectives of emotion from the organismic school, with social perspectives from the interactionist one. Her use of the organismic school is constrained however, limiting understanding of emotion to one of elicitation-expression. In the integration of interactionist theory with Freud, some of the important characteristics about the nature of unconscious emotion and the development or representation of self in the id–ego–superego relationship are lost. Although the significance of interaction in emotion exchanges is clearly identified, in the integration of interactionist theory with organismic approaches, the focus on social factors occludes this importance. This reduces the value of what is arguably Hochschild's most significant contribution to the sociology of emotion, the impact of emotion to, and in, social *interaction*.

These limitations in the conceptualisation of emotion also have implications when Hochschild's understanding of emotional labour is applied to nursing. For, limiting the biological nature of emotion both inhibits understanding about how the physicality of emotion is experienced and managed, and in how it is connected to conscious and unconscious emotion memory. Understanding the nature of emotion elicited in response to the body's flight/fight mechanism as a result of its relationship within the natural environment and in respect to performative skills is important in understanding the role of emotional labour in holistic nursing care. This is particularly relevant if the nature of emotion can render it unmanageable.

In addition, linking Freud's notion of the unconscious too closely with social factors dissipates the value of incorporating the unconscious nature of emotion in its centrality to self and within social interaction – in processes of transference (see Chapter 6). These limitations impact on how the self is theoretically understood within the process of emotion management and emotional labour. Emotional labour in nursing is an interactive and relational exchange. It represents an expression of the nurse's need to care for those individuals who are in need of it. Understanding how emotion is elicited and managed within these emotion exchanges and how it links in with personal and social identity is integral to understanding emotional labour in nursing. In order to develop Hochschild's approach to emotion and understand emotional labour in health care more fully therefore, a way of incorporating a more comprehensive account of the biopsycho nature of emotion with that of the social, without losing the integrity of them, is required. This is explored in Chapter 5.

Vignette 5 'Maxine's rant'

Maxine: I have got home, absolutely distraught, absolutely angry, absolutely stressed. What they did to me this morning was absolutely uncalled for and terrible. I got in – I managed to get there for about two minutes to seven – to find that they had done the allocation. And I just can't believe that they did it. They left me and a bank HCA down A and B who didn't arrive until 8 o'clock, and they had five members of staff down C and D. C and D as I've told you isn't the heavier end of the ward, A and B is. I heard one of the HCAs saying: 'I don't know what she is complaining about.' But they basically knew what they'd done. One of the nurses has a grudge against me, but what really annoyed me was the G grade was there and she let it go on. She knew that the allocation wasn't fair, she knew it. And this is what annoys me, why be a G grade if you are going to let this sort of thing go on. They'd got an E grade, they'd got an acting E, they'd got two senior HCAs and the part-time D grade when she comes on to special that chap. So five members of staff down C and D and they'd left two down A and B [an E grade and a student], which I just don't think is fair and applicable. They've said: 'Oh well, you've got a bank nurse coming in at 8 o'clock', and yes we had a HCA come in at 8 o'clock, so that is three down one end and five down the other. They didn't look at the dependencies, they didn't look at the level of the ward. What they've done is that they will all be laughing and thinking ha, ha, ha! I am fuming and I'm really, really annoyed. *I* wouldn't do it because at the end of the day you are a professional, you don't do those sort of things. I may not like some of the people that I work with, but I would never go out of my way to be that nasty. And it just annoys me. But at the end of the day I do my job to the best of my ability. People on there say, 'Oh, *I'm* a fantastic nurse, *I'm* a great nurse or whatever', because they like blowing their own trumpet or because they like sucking up to the G grade. But what really counts on that ward is the patients. It's a case of, oh well you know, you know . . . ** ! [Splutter, loss of words]

I'm fuming. I've got such a headache. I've just driven home and my head is absolutely splitting, and I know it is with the stress, and I know it's with everything else, and I know I've got myself wound up about it all, but . . . I would just love to tell them . . . I know exactly what they are doing. I know exactly the reason why they've done it. But you don't because you are thinking you've got to work with these people, and you're thinking about the cohesiveness of the ward. But then again, in my mind I'm thinking: 'That's a load of crap.' I should just pull them all in there and tell them what I really do think of them about how cheap and low and nasty and despicable I think they are and how they can call themselves nurses I don't know. And I came that close to getting my bag and my coat and saying: 'Stuff it.' One of them will have to work down A and B when I go, and if the surgical director phones me then I'll say to her, 'I may be black, but I don't have slave or donkey or ass tattooed across the front of my forehead'. I was just so, so *livid* that they did it. I mean I've got a student with me, when am I going to get time to do the drugs with the student? When am I going to get time to work with the HCA? I just think that it is despicable what they did. And the fact that the sister sat there and let them do it, it really, really pissed me off. And sorry about the bad language but it did. And I'm just fed up of the whole thing. And I just felt like saying: 'Well, I might as well go somewhere else where I'll be appreciated'. And then I thought: 'No! That's exactly what those bitches would like: to see me leave'. But I'll see them bloody leave before I go. I know I'm a good nurse and I know what I do is worthwhile and I know that what I do is exceptional and I'm not going to let anybody or anything else put me off that. I nurse to the best of my ability and I think I have a high standard of care and as long as I'm doing that, everyone else can go and get stuffed for all I care.

5   Emotion and personal and social identity

In order to develop Hochschild's notion of emotional labour (including emotion management, surface and deep acting) a more comprehensive approach towards emotion is required. In *Being Human*, Margaret Archer (2000) looks at how emotion connects to personal identity and the acquisition of social identity. She argues that emotions are elicited in response to the relationship individuals have with the natural, material and social world. Striking a balance between different sets of emotions, which emerge in response to these different forms of interaction, is part of the management process. For Archer, this is an ongoing process, mediated through a reflexive 'inner dialogue'. Emotions that emerge as a result of this are intrinsically linked to personal identity, enacted out through social interaction as expressions of social identity. Thus, Archer demonstrates how emotion is intrinsically connected to a sense of personal and social identity without losing the centrality of interaction. In addition, she includes an understanding of the varied ways in which emotion is elicited and experienced in interaction, and which can in itself generate emotion; and that emotion management can be both immediate and extended over a period of time. This chapter introduces Archer's approach to emotion and contrasts it with Hochschild's. It considers how it can be used to develop and complement Hochschild's notion of emotional labour in respect to her understanding of emotion and its relationship with self-identity.

Archer's approach towards emotion

Like Hochschild, Archer's (2000) model of emotion draws together its biopsychosocial nature. Her approach differs in that she separates emotion elicitation from emotion management. She calls emotion elicitation first order emotion and the emotions that emerge from its management, second order emotion. First order emotions are elicited in direct response to interaction with the natural order (the natural environment), the practical order (objects or things) and the social or discursive order (social and cultural context). Second order emotion emerges after first order emotions are reflexively managed, a process which is both cognitively and socially predicated. In this way Archer's analysis allows emotion to be both independent from cognition in its elicitation and co-dependent with it in its management.

Archer sees emotion as essential to conscious awareness which she likens to an inner dialogue. The inner dialogue is the voice inside our head that comments on how and what we are thinking, feeling and experiencing as we go about our daily lives. It is connected therefore to personality, an inner understanding of self. Archer sees emotion as fundamental to the development and nature of 'human being'. She defines emotion from a realist perspective, claiming to avoid reducing emotion to animal essentialism (the debate over whether emotion is innate), subjectivism (which defines it exclusively through social and culture factors), irrationalism (which separates it completely from reason) or cognitivism (which subjects it entirely to cognition).

For Archer, emotions are 'intentional' *'commentaries upon our concerns'*, arising in response to an awareness of what is being engaged with. For example, if I happen to see a spider out of the corner of my eye, I immediately feel fear. This fear represents my perception of spiders as something horrible and threatening, whereas somebody else may not even notice the spider's presence because they do not find them fearful. Or if my partner makes a derogatory remark about me, I would be very upset. However if a perfect stranger did, I would probably respond with indifference. This is because in comparison to the stranger, my partner's opinion matters to me. Thus, quoting Charles Taylor (1985), Archer suggests that emotions are

> relational to something, which is what gives them their emergent character, and that something is our own concerns which make a situation a matter of non-indifference to a person . . . In identifying the import of a situation we are picking out what in that situation gives the grounds or basis of our feelings, we are not just stating that we experience a certain feeling in this situation.
>
> (Archer 2000: 195)

Her definition of emotion as 'affective modes of awareness' is similar to Hochschild's definition of emotion as a sense. However, her approach differs from Hochschild's in five ways. First, for Archer the situation with which individuals are concerned does not have to be social. Rather, it depends on a *relational* understanding of the situation, which also includes body–environment and material relationships. Second, Hochschild's idea of emotion as a sense is passive, interaction becoming relevant only when social factors become involved. For Archer, interaction is embedded in the relational nature of emotion. Third, Archer allows for different kinds of emotion response because emotion can be elicited as a result of different kinds of interaction (such as interaction with an object, such as a piano). Thus, she allows for more than one emotion to be elicited at a time. Archer defines the different types of emotion elicitation as 'clusters' of emotions.

Hochschild's approach is more dualistic: she implies that in any situation there is the emotion that is really felt, and the one that socially ought to be felt. Fourth, Archer incorporates an awareness of time into the inner dialogue, bringing a sense of movement and trajectory to emotion experience. Hochschild's notion of a prior self only draws on past experience and past emotion work. Thus, she loses a sense of the passage of time in the lack of present and future emotion experience.

Archer summarises her approach like this:

(i)   different clusters of emotions represent commentaries upon our concerns and are emergent from our human relationships with the natural, practical and discursive orders of reality respectively. Matters do not finish here.

(ii)   because of our reflexivity, we review these emotion commentaries, articulate them, monitor them, and transmute them; thus elaborating further upon our emotionality itself.

(iii)   this occurs through the inner conversation which is a ceaseless discussion about the satisfaction of our ultimate concerns and a monitoring of the self and its commitments in relation to the commentaries received.

(Archer 2000: 195)

Finally, for Archer, emotion and emotionality are essential to the emergence and recognition of personal identity because how emotions are managed through the inner dialogue reflects individual concerns, interests and values. Personal identity, however, impacts on, and is entwined with, social identity – allowing for individuality within social roles and obligations. In contrast, Hochschild's self is too defined by internalised social factors, which creates a division within the self when conflict occurs. Overall, for Archer, emotions are relationally emergent and can be autonomous of cognition; they are embodied and can be rationally and irrationally, consciously and unconsciously experienced; they are relational and therefore informative about self to self, to others and about other, and in turn they can affect and be influenced by other emotions and by cognition.

First order emotion

Emotion is elicited as a result of interaction with the natural, practical and social or discursive orders (Table 5.1). The **natural order** focuses on the relationship between the body and the environment.

Emotions convey the import of the natural situation to us. Such emotions are emergent from the relationship between nature's properties and our bodily properties – this of course being a necessary relationship given

Table 5.1 Emotion orders

Emotion order	Relational concern	Emerges in respect to
Natural order	Physical wellbeing	Body–environment relations
Practical order	Performative achievement	Subject–object relations
Social order	Self-worth	Subject–subject relations

Source: Adapted from Archer (2000: 199)

the way the world is constituted, the way we are made and the fact that we have to interact ceaselessly.

(Archer 2000: 201)

Archer's notion of the natural order represents the body's need to protect itself as it interacts with the natural environment. That emotion can be elicited directly through the senses without connecting with cognitive neural pathways as a direct reaction to the natural world (Izard 1984; Zajonc 1984; LeDoux 1996, 1998; Turner and Stets 2005) was discussed in Chapter 3. Archer links this with the ability to experience pain and pleasure, suggesting that emotion memory enables the anticipation of pain or pleasure. The flight/fight response, for example, is an immediate reaction to the possibility of remembered pain, or pleasure. When reaction to 'rapidly changing light gradients, such as those that arise with looming objects' (Zajonc 1984: 119) occurs, through the implicit emotion memory, pain is anticipated and fear is immediately experienced. Thus, fear is directly elicited in response to an imminent threat to the body from the environment. In this situation, emotion elicitation and reaction occurs prior to conscious awareness. Cognitive appraisal occurs subsequently, the degree of response being considered rational or irrational in respect to the degree of the threat. Natural order emotions are therefore, concerned with physical wellbeing and emerge from a body–environment relationship. Archer acknowledges that individuals exist and engage with the natural as well as the social world.

The **practical order** is concerned with performative achievement: emotions elicited in response to the competence and skill individuals (the subject) have with things (the object). Understanding subject–object emotion elicitation is important to understanding emotion in the workplace. Archer links this to how individuals materially provide for their physical needs (food, water, shelter, etc.). In order to do this they require skills, and a fair assessment of their competency of those skills. Archer (2000: 198) suggests that this necessitates a 'performative concern' that is 'unavoidably part of our inevitable practical engagement with the world of material culture . . . which [is] historically, cross culturally and socially varied'. In other words, everyone has to learn to earn their keep whether they are a member of the nomadic Innu tribe living off the land using hunting skills, a flight attendant working in the airline industry or a nurse working for the NHS, for 'dealing with the practical world is universal' (Archer 2000: 198).

Emotions associated with the practical order are 'frustration, boredom and depression on the one hand, and satisfaction, joy, exhilaration and euphoria on the other' (Archer 2000: 212). These emotions are important because they reflect the degree to which individuals are skilled or competent at various activities. These emotions truly reflect the self because they are elicited from the relationship between the subject (self) and objects. The object is inanimate and therefore cannot lie. Thus, drawing on Archer's example of the concert pianist, however much an individual may desire to become a concert pianist, unless they have the necessary skill and ability to do so, they cannot manipulate their emotions through deep acting for example, to make it so. Unless the ability is real, feelings of satisfaction and joy when playing the piano cannot be elicited, only feelings of frustration. Emotions elicited from the practical order, therefore are directly linked to self-identity because they reinforce through positive or negative feedback, information about the individual's skills and abilities to themselves, in a way that cannot be fabricated. In respect to personal and social identity, this can be the difference between playing the piano as a hobby, teaching it or being a concert pianist. However, as Archer (2000: 210) points out, judgements about skill and competency are not universally accurate as 'people can deceive themselves, thinking they are better than they are at a given activity'. However, if the individual lies about their ability in order to gain *social* recognition, Archer argues that the emotions elicited from this come from subject–subject relationships represented in the social or discursive order and not the practical one.

The relationship between the kind of knowledge characteristic of practical achievement and the emotions that emerge from it, therefore, are closely linked. The kind of knowledge linked to practical order emotions is encoded through bodily skills. It is habitual tacit knowledge, enacted without conscious awareness that has been directly translated into language. It is not unconscious, however, because it is possible to think about it if necessary. On the whole, feelings are sufficient to keep the individual informed about how well they are performing. For example, having learnt to drive we do not think about the mechanics of driving every time we get into the car. Our body remembers the actions we need to take. However, if we stall the car we might feel momentarily frustrated and apply some conscious thought to getting it going again. Emotions in the practical order therefore, are relational to performative concerns, linked to tacit or pre-reflexive knowledge and skill and contribute to personal identity and emerging social identity. This is immensely important in understanding emotion in the workplace, which often brings the two together, suggesting that an inclusion of subject–object understanding in the elicitation of emotion and the properties that emerge from it could reveal new insights into the purpose of emotional labour and how it relates to personal identity and social identity, satisfaction and dissatisfaction.

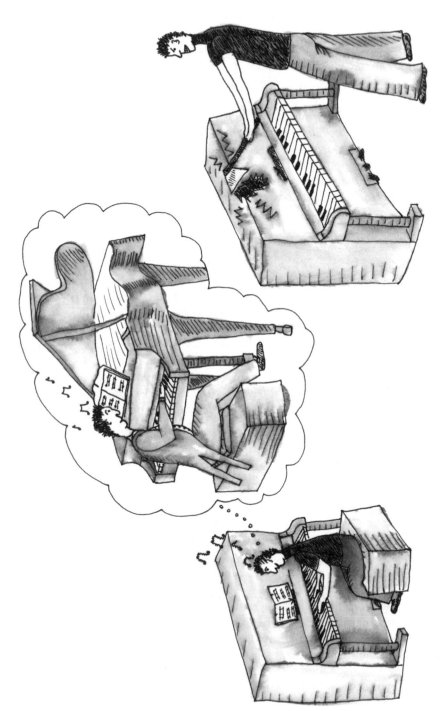

'The concert pianist'

The **social or discursive order** of emotion is concerned with subject–subject relationships: the relationships that individuals have with other people and social institutions. Emotions, such as shame, remorse, pride, envy, jealousy and guilt, elicited from the discursive order are related to self-worth. These emotions are intrinsically social:

> These are *not socially constructed* by the social imposition and individual appropriation of emotional labelling, but rather are *socially constituted properties which are emergent from the internal relationship between the subject's concerns and society's normativity*. Their emergence is thus dependent upon three factors: our subject status in society, the receipt of moral evaluations from the social order and the conjunction between our personal concerns and the nature of society's norms.
>
> (Archer 2000: 215, my emphasis)

Archer's understanding of the social or discursive order is similar to Hochschild's (1983). Like Hochschild, she identifies the importance of the internalisation of social concerns and factors in the ownership of emotion. However, unlike Hochschild, Archer does not see the definition or 'codification' of emotion as being dependent on social factors. Thus, they are not fixed or 'reified'. She suggests that understanding emotions elicited from the social order is subjective. This is because the individual has to engage with, or be concerned about, the social activity in which they are involved for the emotions to be elicited in the first instance. In this way, emotions elicited from the social order are fundamentally related to the subject's self-worth because they are social aspects that they consider important to them.

> Generically, the most important of our social concerns is our self worth which is vested in certain projects (career, family, community, club or church) whose success or failure we take as vindicating our worth or damaging it. It is *because we have invested ourselves in these social projects that we are susceptible of emotionality in relation to society's evaluation of our performance in these roles*. Our behaviour is regulated by hopes and fears, that is anticipations of social approbation/disapprobation.
>
> (Archer 2000: 219, my emphasis)

This allows for choice and for the personality of individuals to emerge and become part of society, whereas Hochschild's feeling rules tend to be more generalised. Thus, as noted earlier, Hochschild applies them to all individuals, indiscriminately – in fact in Hochschild's theory, this is a necessary part in defining and labelling emotion. Archer, on the other hand, directly makes socially constructed feeling rules optional to individuals because for them to matter, the subject needs to have a relationship with them. She comments: 'normative discourse is about the moral evaluation of our comportment as acceptable or unacceptable . . . and is not about labelling emotional states or about subjects' appropriation of labels' (Archer 2000: 218). This allows for differences in the values that individuals place on their own and others actions, thereby allowing for individuality. Archer's analysis shows how emotion is intimately connected with personal identity in conjunction with social identity where there is shared expectation and understanding about the roles held. Thus, while all nurses might share a common role and identity represented in feeling rules and emotional labour, in each individual those roles are mixed with other ones such as family, community, club or church. The intertwining of personal identity with social identity can moderate the importance of others' approval or disapproval of their role performance. Thus in nursing, emotional labour holds varying degrees of importance among nurses. By making emotion relational and therefore personal to each individual, Archer reflects Goffman's focus on deviance from social norms influencing behaviour more readily than Hochschild does. Archer writes:

> It is our own definitions of what constitutes our self worth that determines which normative evaluations matter enough for us to be emotional about them. In strict parallel, what we are emotional about also makes it possible to constitute the good life in society for particular people. Thus, for the emergence of social emotions, it is not sufficient that society has a normative register and that its members continuously pass a stream of evaluations on the comportment of fellow subjects: in addition we have to be parties to these social norms.
>
> (Archer 2000: 219–220)

Using Archer's approach it is also possible to see how private and public emotion can be distinguished in respect to an individual's personal identity and autonomy of choice, rather than being a difference in place, as they are for Hochschild (see Chapter 1). This is because personal and social identities are held in tandem. This distinction is more realistic than Hochschild's because what individuals deem private and personal may depend on the kind of relationships they have with others, which can vary irrespective to the place in which interaction occurs. Thus, the distinction between private and public is really one of ownership and relationship of self rather than one of place.

In empirical research, Archer's approach also sheds light on how emotion can be observed and inquired about in respect to what aspects of their emotional lives individuals consider to be private in the workplace. This is important when seeking to determine what is important to groups, such as nurses and to individuals within those groups.

Archer's notion of emotions that are elicited through the social or discursive order enables a more comprehensive understanding of individuality and the differences that exist between people despite their similar social circumstances. She also accounts for individual choice and autonomy. This is essential because it shows how individuals or groups of individuals can affect social change irrespective of social constraints. Emotions often provide motivation to such action. However, arguably, she does allow too great a freedom to individuals. Hochschild (1983) notes how emotion can be shaped and even reinterpreted as a result of interaction. Although she does not fully develop this (see Chapter 4), it is an important point. Individuals do not always have a choice about the social activity in which they are involved, or their place and role in it. These can bring with them social expectations and responsibilities, which can be the measures others judge by. For example, if an individual is new to a role, they may allow the values and judgements of others to influence their own values, or even their perceptions about their performance. Equally, while one individual may not set a huge store by a particular role, while performing it others might, and their judgement might impact on them irrespective of their personal choice. This is where the passage of time can become important. Personal and social identity changes and develops throughout life. In her notion of second order emotion, Archer is able to introduce a time trajectory into the individual's emotional commentary.

First order emotion in 'Maxine's rant' (Vignette 5)

The natural order

The natural order is most readily represented in 'The scrotal drain' (Vignette 3), where the patient experiences high levels of anxiety in anticipation of pain. This anxiety emerges because he is concerned about his physical wellbeing. In Vignette 5, however, there is a visceral response to the emotions that Maxine experiences. She comments that she has a 'splitting headache' which she knows is due to stress. It is arguable that the environment in which she has been working is a hostile one. This hostility keeps her emotionally alert throughout the shift.

The practical order

In Vignette 5, Maxine comments that she is a good nurse who has a high standard of care that she carries out to the best of her ability. This suggests she experiences feelings of satisfaction due to her professional competencies and skills.

The social order

The emotions of anger and humiliation which run throughout Vignette 5 are elicited as a result of Maxine's social interaction with her colleagues.

ANGER

Maxine sees the distribution of the workload as being unfair because she believes that it should be based on the dependency levels of each end of the ward. These levels are assessed at the end of each shift according to the degree of every patient's care dependency needs. Score 4 is the highest dependency and requires the most input from the nursing staff, while score 1 is the lowest and requires the least. Maxine believes that the distribution of staff is unfair because she has the greatest number of high dependency patients, consequently her workload is higher. This elicits anger in Maxine.

HUMILIATION

Maxine interprets this division of the labour as an act of aggression designed to humiliate her in front of the G grade ward sister. She perceives it as a rejection of her as an individual. She identifies that one of the nurses has a grudge against her, and that she knows this nurse is laughing at her behind her back. She is hurt by the nurse's actions. It hurts because she wants to be accepted by her colleagues.

Archer's notion of first order emotion is useful in identifying what emotions are present. It also illustrates how these emotions reflect something that is intrinsic to the individual experiencing them in relation to the context in which they are interacting.

Second order emotion

The elicitation of first order emotion is only part of the emotional experience. Archer suggests that an emotional commentary materialises as the emotions from the natural, practical and social order emerge and collide. For 'nothing guarantees that the three sets of emotions dovetail harmoniously, and therefore it follows that the concerns to which they relate cannot all be promoted without conflict arising between them' (Archer 2000: 220). Unless a person 'is otherwise incapable of reflection' (2000: 221), this is where reflexivity or cognitive appraisal enters into the process. Striking a balance between different sets of emotions, and the emotions that emerge from this process is what Archer terms second order emotion. Second order emotion is achieved through a reflexive 'inner conversation' from which an individual's personal identity is shaped. Archer (2000: 222) defines reflexivity as 'our ability to reflect upon our emotionality itself, to transform it and consequently to reorder priorities within our emotional sets'.

The internal conversation involves a series of progressive articulations and rearticulations – the 'inner dialogue' between 'I', 'you' and 'me', which happens over a period of time. Here, individuals conduct an inner conversation with themselves commenting on, and making sense of how they feel in respect to what they are engaging with. For example, I might wake up one morning feeling 'strange', unsure of why (first order emotions). Then I might observe to myself:

> Well, I am feeling a bit nervous because I have an exam today but while I am anxious that I do well in it, I am looking forward to finishing and celebrating afterwards. I feel strange therefore because I am nervous and excited at the same time.

Through this inner dialogue, I have articulated what those emotions are, becoming conversant with my emotion state, able to define and understand it. These understood emotions are second order emotions. Archer sees this as a process moving from the elicitation of first order to second order emotion through the inner dialogue. This process is represented in Table 5.2.

Because the inner dialogue is individual, it is unique to the self. Hochschild (1983) develops 'the self' in her notion of deep acting in which she juxtaposes Freud's ego, with Mead's 'I' and 'me'. However, in order to integrate the two she makes social factors primary, and her self divides into 'true' and 'false'. For Archer, the emergence of personal identity is linked to the inner dialogue. She avoids creating a false and true self partly because she separates emotion elicitation from its management and partly because she juxtaposes Freud's notion of ego with Charles Peirce's idea of internal conversation (Peirce 1998: para. 6). By excluding the id and superego, Archer avoids ontological difficulties in integrating psychological 'unconscious' perspectives with sociological ones. She appears to succeed because primary emotions – which

Table 5.2 The inner dialogue

Elicitation of first order emotions

——————————————▶

      Articulation and rearticulation of the inner dialogue

      ——————————————▶

            Elaboration of second order emotions

            ——————————————▶

Source: Adapted from Archer (2000: 227)

may never be attached to conscious awareness – are included as first order emotions. Arguably such emotions may equate with those expressed by the id, while the inner dialogic process, which represents concerns that the individual invests themselves in – and therefore has a moral component – could equate to the role of the superego.

Peirce looks at different phases of the ego in dialogue, relating it to the inner conversation between 'you', 'I' and 'me'. Archer sees this conversation as being part of the articulation–rearticulation process. For example, a conversation might reflect a process such as 'I feel so and so because this just happened to me, but if I think about it in relation to that, you might feel differently later, don't you think?' Peirce suggests that the 'I' of the present can address the future self through the 'you' by criticising, ordering or anticipating in relation to past experience, present or future events. The 'me' (which is non-Meadean) represents a more overall sense of self held in the emotion memory: 'the "me" is all the former "Is" who have moved down the time line of future, past and present' (Archer 2000: 229). The dialogue directly links emotions to rational cognitive processes and together they comment on the activities the individual is involved in. The emotions that emerge as a consequence of this dialogue are second order emotions.

The inner dialogue

Archer identifies three phases of the inner dialogic process: discernment, deliberation and dedication. In the **discernment phase**, the 'I', 'you' and 'me' work together to identify what concerns them most when confronted with choices. This is achieved by the 'I' appealing or aspiring in its commentary about the present situation to the 'you' in the future. For example, the nurse dealing with the vomiting patient might be thinking, 'I wish I could deal with this better' or 'Come on Catherine, you can do better than this'. These appeals or aspirations are judged by the 'you' in light of the retrospective 'me', based on memory: 'I wouldn't feel so bad about how I have handled the care of this patient if I had anticipated the likelihood of their being sick and given an antiemetic.' Discernment therefore is an exploration of possible actions to change, based on reproach and challenges. In itself, discernment is inconclusive and always changing in response to the present situation; it achieves its aim in highlighting concerns, and the process moves forward into deliberation.

The **deliberation phase** of the conversation finds the 'I' or the 'you' directly asking 'How much do you care about it?' and 'How far will you go?' In essence it sets about identifying the cost of the enterprise. So, the nurse caring for the vomiting patient might ask how far she should go in her action to prevent vomiting. Should she give all her patients antiemetics? This action could cost valuable time in assessing the likelihood of nausea and vomiting, and in identifying, preparing and administering the correct antiemetic. Giving an antiemetic could also mask an important symptom, or in giving antiemetics indiscriminately, detract from the satisfaction she gets from dealing with her patients as individuals. These questions posed together by the 'I' and answered by the 'you', drawing on the experience of the 'me', 'reprioritise their concerns, demoting and promoting, cutting the coat as the emotional cloth allows' (Archer 2000: 237). When the concerns have been raised and anticipated (discernment) and the cost to the individual of different courses of action have been both emotionally and cognitively questioned (deliberation), the inner conversation leads on to the dedication phase.

The **dedication phase** involves prioritising the first order emotions and coming to a working balance which can be lived with. Having added up the balance and come to a conclusion over the degree of commitment, the individual then determines the *overall cost* of the decided course of action in relation to their self-worth and self-integrity. For example, can the nurse sustain such a high degree of concern for every potentially vomiting patient? Will exhibiting such concern cost her her place in the peer group? Is she sure that this degree of care is essential to her self-worth? Should she continue in nursing if such attention to detail is required for every patient and their possible care needs?

The inner dialogue in 'Maxine's rant' (Vignette 5)

Discernment phase

First, Maxine identifies her first order emotions: 'I have got home, absolutely distraught, absolutely angry, absolutely stressed.' In discerning why this matters to her, Maxine's 'I' appeals to herself, 'I just can't believe that they did it', and she identifies the unfairness of it exclaiming: '*I* wouldn't do it.' She discerns what it is they have done to her 'me' – an appeal to her continuous sense of self. 'They left me and a bank HCA down A and B.' This is unfair because 'as I've told you, [it] isn't the heavier end of the ward'.

Having discerned why she is so angry, Maxine works out what they have done to her 'me'. Here her inner dialogue bounces between her 'I' and 'you':

> They didn't look at the dependencies, they didn't look at the level of the ward. What they've done [*to me*] is that they will all be laughing and thinking ha, ha, ha! *I* am fuming and *I'm* really, really annoyed. *I* wouldn't do it because at the end of the day *you* are a professional, *you* don't do those sorts of things.

She is also discerning why the other nurses have acted in this way. What were they hoping to achieve. It is not just an unfair allocation of the workload; it is an act of aggression designed to make a point. Maxine discerns why they have done that to her 'me': 'One of the nurses has a grudge against *me*, but what really annoyed *me* was the G grade was there and she let it go on. She knew that the allocation wasn't fair, she knew it.'

She notes that even though one of the nurses has a grudge against her these actions are still not justified:

> *You* don't do those sort of things. *I* may not like some of the people that *I* work with, but *I* would never go out of *my* way to be that nasty. And it just annoys *me*. But at the end of the day *I* do *my* job to the best of *my* ability. People on there say, 'Oh, I'm a fantastic nurse, I'm a great nurse or whatever', because they like blowing their own trumpet or because they like sucking up to the G grade. But what really counts on that ward is the patients. It's a case of, oh well *you* know, *you* know . . . ** !

By giving Maxine a higher workload they place her in a position where she may not be able to perform her duties properly. This would make Maxine seem less competent than her colleagues. However, Maxine discerns this bullying strategy.

Deliberation phase

Having discerned what she is feeling and why she is feeling it, Maxine moves on to deliberate how much this matters to her, and how far can she go in the kind of response she makes. To do this her 'I' questions, and her 'you' responds:

> *I* would just love to tell them . . . *I* know exactly what they are doing. *I* know exactly the reason why they've done it. But *you* don't because *you* are thinking *you've* got to work with these people, and *you're* thinking about the cohesiveness of the ward. But then again, in *my* mind *I'm* thinking: 'That's a load of crap.' *I* should just pull them all in there and tell them what *I* really do think of them about how cheap and low and nasty and despicable *I* think they are and how they can call themselves nurses *I* don't know. And *I* came that close to getting *my* bag and *my* coat and saying: 'Stuff it.' One of them will have to work down A and B when *I* go, and if the surgical director phones *me* then *I'll* say to her, '*I* may be black, but *I* don't have slave or donkey or ass tattooed across the front of *my* forehead'.

Here, as Maxine's internal conversation deliberates on her response she also draws on the experience of her 'me' and her emotion memory, linking the bullying of the other nurses to racial issues. The deliberation phase continues as she considers what the effect of this action might be:

> And *I* just felt like saying, 'Well, *I* might as well go somewhere else where *I'll* be appreciated'. And then *I* thought: 'No! That's exactly what those bitches would like: to see *me* leave'. But *I'll* see them bloody leave before *I* go.

Through the deliberation phase she realises that leaving will not bring about the desired effect and would be too costly to her.

Dedication phase

Here, practical first order emotions come into the dialogue, and she realises that not only is she a good nurse and this brings her satisfaction, but also this is important to her self-worth because she believes in the value of it. Thus, as she moves into the dedication phase, she considers the overall cost this course of action might bring, and reconsiders how this might affect her integrity of self: '*I* know *I'm* a good nurse and *I* know what *I* do is worthwhile and *I* know that what *I* do is exceptional and *I'm* not going to let anybody or anything else put *me* off that.'

And her inner dialogue concludes: '*I* nurse to the best of *my* ability and *I* think *I* have a high standard of care and as long as *I'm* doing that, everyone else can go and get stuffed for all *I* care.'

Her inner dialogue has brought her to the realisation that her sense of self is strong enough in its purpose to sustain the act of aggression. She moves into second order emotion, and decides she does not care. Through her inner dialogue, Maxine has worked through emotions elicited from the first order, and in balancing them out decides that her anger and humiliation are less relevant than her feelings of satisfaction. Thus, despite the act of aggression by the other nurses in which they imply that if she cannot cope she is not a good nurse, by giving her a heavier workload, Maxine realises that this is not the case. She therefore dismisses her anger and humiliation secure in the knowledge that she is a capable and good nurse. Despite the intensity of the emotions and the awfulness of situation, her emotion work enables the realisation that it has not sufficiently challenged her sense of integrity and social identity as a nurse because her personal identity is robust enough to sustain the attack.

Contrasting Hochschild and Archer

Archer's differentiation between first and second order emotion offers the more comprehensive account of emotion. The distinction between the natural, practical and social or discursive order in first order emotion enables the identification of different emotions as they are elicited in relation to something. Emotions express the relations individuals have with the world around them, and which they are an integral part of. In this sense emotions communicate to them, and to others, a sense of what is being interacted with (Burkitt 1997). The separation of emotion elicitation from its management acknowledges that reflexive management does not always take place. Thus Archer accounts for the experience and expression of emotion as being both independent from conscious cognitive process and connected with it. Consequently, her approach encompasses the organismic nature of emotion and integrates it with emotion's cognitive nature more successfully than Hochschild's.

Archer's theory of the emergence of personal identity from second order emotionality also offers a more complex and integrated way of understanding how the ego might mediate between differently elicited emotions than Hochschild's theory. Hochschild's notion of deep acting is limited to its specific purpose in carrying out emotional labour as part of a socially defined identity, reducing the ego to mediating between the real self and the self-induced self through deep acting. Thus, according to Hochschild's notion of deep acting, the nurse dealing with the vomiting patient may suppress feelings of disgust triggered by the vomiting, and by using her imagination or emotion memory evoke feelings of empathy and concern in order to care for her patient. The emotion management that occurs here is dualistic in nature; one emotion is elicited, then suppressed, and another is expressed in its place.

Archer's approach allows for a more complex emotion experience than this. The nurse dealing with the vomiting patient experiences different emotions elicited from the first order. In the natural order *disgust* is elicited at the vomit (body–environment), motivating the nurse to change that environment by cleaning it up and also cleaning up the patient and trying to prevent the event from occurring again. In the practical order *satisfaction* or *dissatisfaction* is elicited according to how well the nurse deals with the situation (subject–object). In the social order emotions concerned with whether she in fact cares about the vomiting patient (subject–subject) are elicited. If she does care, she may feel *guilty, ashamed* or *remorseful* for not anticipating the likelihood of the patient vomiting, or she may take *pride* in how she interacts with and cares for her patient in the event of her vomiting, gaining a degree of self-worth from how she is seen to be accomplishing her work. Through her inner dialogue, the nurse evaluates the balance between being practically efficient, leaving the patient to be cleaned up by the HCA, and going to the treatment room to prepare the antiemetic and informing the doctor of the event, as opposed to being the one who cleans and reassures the patient. On the other hand, the emotions elicited from the natural order may result in her avoiding the situation; she may not gain satisfaction in the practical achievement of dealing with the situation or her self-worth may not be concerned with how other people might judge her as caring or non-caring, and in reality, balancing these emotions through the inner dialogue, she may gain satisfaction and self-worth by delegating the responsibility of cleaning the patient to the HCA and getting on with an entirely different aspect of care which, to her, has a higher priority. Thus, the nurse experiences and manages several emotions. In addition, Archer's account allows for different individual interpretations to the event of a patient vomiting and therefore, differences in choice of action according to the nurses' personal identity rather than representing simple deviance from a social norm as Hochschild suggests.

Second order emotionality is directly connected to and integrated in the emergence of personal identity. Unlike social identity, it is not formed solely through constraining cultural and structural norms; rather it is fundamentally linked to self-integrity and personal choice. Through this link it is possible to discern that personal choice and action are related to individual personality whilst they are still also made within socially constrained settings with their prescribed structures and roles. For example, in Chapter 2 Paris and Amelia in Vignettes 1 and 2 respectively had different approaches to, and interpretations of, emotional labour. Second, linking emotions with personal identity, thus enabling voluntary choice, accounts for emotion which motivates actions that are not constrained by cultural or structural norms. Such actions have the potential to challenge and change social norms, values and systems, like system failures and technological advancements can. Thus, Archer directly relates emotion to personal identity and to social praxis. This is important, because emotional labour in nursing is constantly developing in response to changes in the delivery of nursing care (Olesen and Bone 1998), necessitating a means by which this can be identified and understood.

Hochschild does however set out to deal with social norms and values and the action of individuals from within social identities and prescribed roles. Feeling rules are essential to this. Thus, Archer's evaluation can take place only if social norms, values or feeling rules have previously been identified. The example of the nurse above is based on feeling rules that suggest nurses should directly care for physically ill people, and that the value of that care is part of their role and identity.

Archer's inner dialogue is entirely cognitive, excluding unconscious emotion. Although she acknowledges that not everybody can (because they are too young and have not fully developed a sense of identity, or because they always react to first order emotions) move from first order emotion to second order emotionality, she does not allow for those who repress or suppress their emotion. In fact, Archer notes that because Freud's analysis of the unconscious includes 'the dynamics of repression and projection'

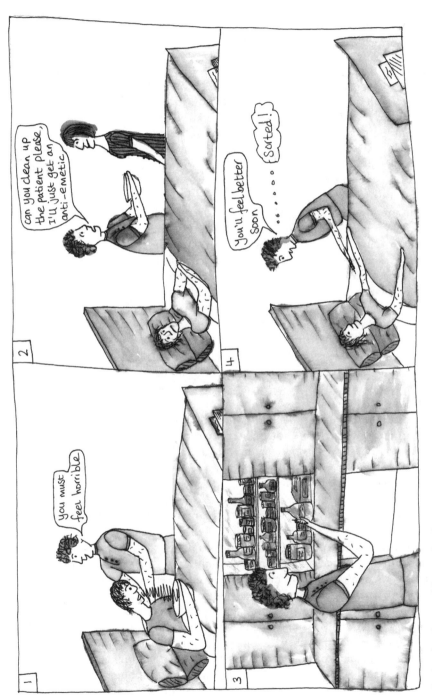

'Caring for the vomiting patient'

(Archer 2000: 194) which are explicit to personal psychology and not social interaction, they cannot be included in Peirce's notion of the inner dialogue. Hochschild's incorporation of suppression and repression, however, shows how essential they are in understanding the nature of emotion management especially in how emotion is enacted through surface and deep acting. This suggests that both suppression and repression can be understood within social interactionist frameworks. Hochschild's suggestion of emotion suppression as a means to an end also offers an important insight when the reflexive balancing act fails, effecting what Hochschild identifies as the authenticity of emotion and the real self, and what for Archer would presumably be a cost to the individual's personal integrity and therefore, their sense of self-worth. Thus, unconscious, repressed and suppressed emotions constitute a surprising omission in Archer's work. For example, the nurse may choose through her inner dialogue to help the vomiting patient practically by preparing and administering an antiemetic, not because it elicits satisfaction, but because she fears the disapprobation of her peers if she stays and cleans up the patient. She chooses this action because of emotions elicited from the social order which relate to her self-worth in her own eyes and that of her peers. However, this can also elicit guilt and shame because it is in conflict with emotions that are integral to her self-worth as a person who would prefer to care for the patient's immediate needs before administering the antiemetic, thereby eliciting feelings of pride from the social order and greater satisfaction from the practical order. However, in choosing this action she would experience feelings of guilt (because her action takes longer) and shame (because her action is different from the peer group and therefore she is excluded) in relation to her performance in the eyes of her peers – feelings she might consequently suppress. Archer does note that at the end of the discernment, deliberation and dedication phases, the nurse still has to ask whether her choice is worth it overall, but does not go on to comment that if there is no resolution to a conflict, what emotions might be elicited directly from that conflict, or suppressed or repressed because of the balancing act.

Hochschild's notion of deep acting also highlights the role of inducing or exhorting emotion through use of the individual's emotion memory or imagination. For Hochschild this is linked to external social factors, but the process of inducement or exhortation is achieved through internal psychological processes that may actually bypass or exclude first order emotion elicitation or take precedence over the emergence of second order emotion from the inner dialogue. First order emotions therefore maybe unconscious, elicited through implicit emotion memory. However, Archer does not include how unconscious emotion may impact on second order emotion or affect the inner dialogue. One of Hochschild's strengths is her acknowledgement of unconscious and repressed components of emotion. Although she limits her use of Freud by changing his original meaning when she integrates him with social interactionist perspectives, she does show how unconscious emotion can impact on emotion experience, management and expression. By restoring Freud's original meaning and incorporating his notion of repression and projection with Archer's first and second order emotion connected through the inner dialogue, Hochschild's notion of unconscious emotion management and the repression of emotion can be developed.

This is not without difficulty. However, some of this is due to Archer's conceptualisation of the inner dialogic process. For example, she does not allow for the possibility that an individual may go through the inner dialogic process without second order emotion emerging because some first order emotions, such as anger or grief, may dominate in a way that an individual cannot control or manage. Here it is possible that an individual becomes trapped in a constant conscious and reflexive dialogue, unable to suppress or move away from the dominant emotion, causing further emotions and mental anguish. This difficulty arises due to the linear process of Archer's inner dialogue and because she does not account for unconscious emotions being misinterpreted by the conscious mind.

For example, Archer's model of second order emotionality emerging through the inner dialogue is one of process, always moving from the present into the future. There is an assumption therefore that through the dialogue, reflexivity always moves forward. However, in her conceptualisation of the 'me', which represents a sense of continuous identity, in drawing on past experiences and projecting them into the present and future, it is possible for the emotion dialogue to become circular, or to rebound from the present or future, back into a past conflict or dilemma (see Figure 5.1). This would allow for unresolved emotion memories to impact, use of emotion memory

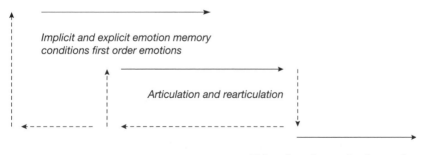

Key:

Archer's time flow ⟶

Negative feedback ----→

Figure 5.1 Negative feedback in the inner dialogue

to exhort or induce and for implicit emotion memory to unconsciously influence the dialogic process. However, because Archer's inner dialogue is processual, the passage of time illustrating emotion trajectory, is incorporated. This is important to retain because emotion management is not entirely based on past experiences; it is ongoing, representing a continuous understanding of self that has a past, present and future. A sense of conflict, and a sense of process, therefore, is a necessary part of the inner dialogue. This could be represented by incorporating a negative feedback loop within the articulation and rearticulation phase of the inner dialogue (Figure 5.1).

Integrating Hochschild and Archer in analysing 'Maxine's rant' (Vignette 5)

Maxine was the victim of bullying, when the other nurses allocated her to A and B bay with only one HCA and a student, while five members of staff were working in C, D and E bay. The emotional impact of this was huge. The allocation took place before 7am, and eight hours later, after working a full shift, their actions still have the power to make her furious. The events at the beginning of the shift defined and made real all subsequent interactions during the shift. In order to successfully carry out her nursing duties, Maxine would have had to *suppress* these feelings, which constitutes surface acting. Although to us it is obvious that Maxine has been humiliated, Maxine *induces* anger, to minimise her feelings of shame – although there is also acknowledgement of being humiliated. The reason this humiliation was so spectacular was because, like Maxine, these were senior nurses and their actions were upheld by the G grade colluding with them. This ensured that Maxine was made to accept the lowest place among them. Behind Maxine's anger, therefore, is shame. The strength of her anger however, visibly grows throughout the extract as she deliberately stokes and fuels it.

Maxine directly exhorts feelings from past experiences to sustain and project her feelings of injustice and evoke feelings of anger and resentment. She says: 'I may be black, but I don't have slave or donkey or ass tattooed across the front of my forehead'. This reaffirms her sense of identity drawn from her cultural heritage as a black person. Her emotion memory in this case is used not to create false feelings (Hochschild) but to exhort, sustain and make sense of the feelings she already has (her 'me'). Being ill-treated just because one is black is widely considered unjustified. There is a similarity, therefore, in the unfairness of being ill-treated due to prejudice and being given an unfair allocation because one is not liked. Invoking this memory and the emotions associated with it, fuels the sense of injustice, indignation and resentment at such treatment.

Here, Maxine consciously exhorts and transfers remembered associations with racial prejudice. Some of this process may be unconscious – in that she unconsciously draws feelings associated with such situations, and in doing so *becomes* aware of them, making it a more conscious process. It is also likely that there are unconscious emotions related to ill-treatment that are similarly painful, but not necessarily directly related to prejudicial treatment. As a result of its moral connotation, associating such experiences with racial prejudice may be less painful, allowing the self (in the present) to avoid and protect itself from the painful self-acknowledgement of negative characteristics.

Maxine also uses her imagination to play out a fantasy scenario when she imagines taking the offending nurses into the office and telling them what she really thinks of them, and in the imaginary act of leaving the ward throws all the work they expect her to do into their hands. In this fantasy she both induces and works through her anger, so that subsequently she can display a 'don't care' attitude and dismiss those nurses' actions when she works with them in the future. Her emotion management is preparatory work for later surface and deep acting that projects a different emotion attitude to the one her emotion work is currently inducing. While she uses her imagination to achieve this, therefore, the emotions she evokes through this process are not the ones which she expresses in deep acting carried out in her interactions with this group of nurses. Instead they are part of her private inner dialogue that empowers subsequent emotional labour. Her deep acting does not displace real emotion, rather it works through and expresses it in order to transcend it and restore her own sense of self.

Vignette 5 illustrates how imagination and emotion memory project into the inner dialogue, and how in the articulation and rearticulation process, they are central to empowering personal identity. This is necessary because the allocation of Maxine to A and B bay by the other nurses was a direct statement of power as well as an assertion of status and place. Maxine perceives this as a slur on her personal identity. However, her confidence and pride in her role and abilities as a nurse are not dented because she knows that it is because they dislike her. She notes several times that it is not because she is a bad nurse that she is being bullied, it is because of who she is, and what she is perceived to stand for. In her emotion commentary, this gives her a sense of self-righteousness and enables her to draw on her moral integrity in contrast to the 'lack' of moral integrity of the others. Thus, Maxine's inner dialogue reflects her sense of self in values that matter to her. In this, she relates her moral feelings to her own sense of self, empowering her belief and reinforcing those feelings in the process. Thus, in her final statement she decides to rub their noses in her continued presence on the ward as an assertion of that empowerment, because in the belief that her nursing skills are beyond reproach, she sees her actions as justified and morally acceptable in contrast to theirs. This acknowledgement limits the power the others can exert over her because she does not lose confidence in her abilities.

In the fantasy scenario, she acknowledges the kind of emotional bullying she is the victim of by reversing it in the threat to leave the ward, thereby asserting their need of her in her role as a senior nurse. Thus, in her fantasy, she reverses the balance of power between herself and the others without changing their original actions and therefore, their unjustified stance. Her anticipation of her future interactions with these nurses is not conciliatory or submissive. Rather, through her inner dialogue, second order emotions emerge which empower her to maintain her sense of individuation in the face of the others' rejection of her. This empowerment motivates her choice to continue working on the ward and to gain satisfaction from doing so.

Her sustained sense of self is then acted out the next day in her emotion work. Her diary entry for the following shift starts with:

> I've had a good shift. It was very, very busy. Still short in numbers down in A and B and it is still quite heavy. I had one medical emergency, with a patient who had extended his CVA [cerebral vascular accident] and his wife was quite distraught.

Her entire attitude towards the quantity of the work has changed and she makes no further reference in the diary to the allocation incident at all. Her emotion management enables her to choose not to react. Thus, her comment that she is a good nurse and what she does is worthwhile and that she is not going to let anybody influence that is borne out.

Conclusion

Use of Archer's approach is valuable because it enables a greater focus on emotion itself. Because emotions are considered as commentaries on concerns and because they are relational, it is emotion that informs the self as it continuously interacts with the natural, material and social world. Likewise, emotion management is driven by the relational, interactive and commentary nature of emotion and is therefore understood within this relationship. A sense of self emerges through an interrelated emotion and cognitive commentary that is also relational and interactive. This approach towards emotion can be used to develop Hochschild's notion of emotion management and consequently, in understanding and developing the relationship between emotion and emotional labour in nursing.

For example, in Chapter 2 (p. 48), four distinct differences between the emotional labour of nurses and that of flight attendants were identified (see also Table 3.1, page 53). Archer's approach towards emotion is useful here. First, Archer's notion of first order emotions includes interaction with the natural and practical order. Nursing care is often concerned with the physical body and clinical nursing skills are performative in nature. The importance of the natural and practical orders often takes precedence over the social, as seen in Vignette 1, 'Half measures'. These components of nursing care therefore need to be included in an understanding of emotional labour that is holistic.

Second, interaction is always ongoing, as is Archer's inner dialogue; emotion management develops in response to ongoing interaction over time. In Vignette 2, 'Alix's dad', Amelia's relationship with Alix's dad developed over several months. Her emotional labour reflects not only each separate interaction, but also an ongoing, developing relationship. This also connects to a further difference; that emotional labour in nursing is interactive and *relational*. Fundamental to this is that that relationship is predicated on the interaction between at least two people who all have a sense of personal identity in respect to their social one. Archer's approach facilitates a more comprehensive understanding of the nature of emotional labour here.

Third, emotional labour is needed by patients because they are vulnerable; it is implicated therefore, in mediating power and trust. Archer's approach adds important elements in understanding this point. This is because she sees emotions as a commentary on the individuals' concerns, which are therefore implicated in interaction. Thus, the emotions *of those being cared for* are also relevant to the analysis, because they arise because of the situations they are in. It is because of their ill health that they require care in the first place. They are frightened, angry, humiliated, shamed or in denial because what is happening matters to them. Thus, they are vulnerable. This is the context in which the nurse interacts, appraises and responds. The emotional labour that she carries out therefore, is interactive within this relational context. Thus, it is because emotional labour is interactive and relational that it can be implicated in mediating power and trust within the caring relationship. It is also possible for the nurse to wield power over the vulnerable by withholding emotional labour. Archer's account allows for this too, because emotions are commentaries on individuals concerns, they are linked to personal identity and the choices individuals make in respect to what they consider is important to them.

However, Archer's approach limits understanding of some aspects of the emotional exchange involved in emotional labour. This is because second order emotion emerges as a result of a linear processual inner dialogue, which is entirely cognitive. Thus unresolved conflicts between emotions (past and/ or present), or the impact of unconscious emotions are not included in the inner dialogue. However, because she separates emotion elicitation from its management, within analysis, elicited emotions irrespective of whether the individual experiencing them consciously recognises them, can be identified. With the inclusion of a negative feedback loop in the inner dialogue, Freud's representation of the relationship between the id–ego–superego and the unconscious and Hochschild's notion of emotion exhortation can be tentatively integrated into the analysis here. Thus, Archer's approach towards emotion can be used to develop understanding of the relationship between emotion and emotional labour in nursing due to its focus on emotion and its connection with self-identity.

Part II

Developing emotional labour in nursing

A theoretically informed empirical approach

Vignette 6 'An average shift'

Paula: I have just finished an early shift; it was quite good actually as early shifts go. I had a student with me and two HCAs down my end [A and B]. The student always likes to come and do the drugs. So we check the patient's name band: we have to do it properly when you have a student, so it took a little longer to do the drugs than normal. We hadn't quite finished when the doctors started doing their rounds. The consultant asked the HO [house officer] to get a staff nurse so I had to go round with him. I had to put the drugs back in the lock-up cupboard and go round with the consultant, with the result that some people did not get their 8 o'clock drugs until well after the doctor's round because he had to look at everybody's dressing and then ask me about social problems of one patient, and by the time we had been in all the MRSA rooms, it was quite late.

Meanwhile the HCAs had done the breakfasts and were getting some of the patients out of bed and making the beds. As soon as we finished the doctor's round, the student and I finished the drugs. We then dealt with any pain problems and I then checked the IVs. I then told the rest of the team – namely the other two HCAs – what the consultant had said about the patients. I then had an enquiry from a relative as to why her husband's operation had been cancelled the day before and when she could talk to a doctor to find out when his operation was likely to be. I gave her the number of the consultant's secretary so that she could phone her and make an appointment to see him or one of his team. Then the social worker phoned up and asked about a patient who was going home; as far as I knew everything was in place, but he needed the bottom of his chair raised and this was all we were waiting for, but it was keeping him in a £250 per night bed. After that, I took the student to one side and showed her how to do aseptic technique and made her watch me do a dressing, and then I let her do a dressing and talked her through it and then she helped me with all the other dressings. This takes up time. We then got on with bathing and showering the people that the HCAs hadn't managed to get around to and then we started observations [10am] and then it was our breakfast break.

When we came back, the bed manager was on the ward saying that she had to get six patients in because they had been cancelled before, and asked who we had going home. At that point I didn't know anybody was going home from my end, so I discussed with the staff nurse from the other end and she said that she had three patients going home. We were also on surgical take [emergency admissions] and so this left us very short of beds. The bed manager asked what outliers [non-vascular surgical patients] we had. We had six, so she arranged for two to go to the orthopaedic ward and two to go to another orthopaedic ward and one to go back to a medical ward and one to go to the elderly wing, so that we could get our six patients in and still leave ourselves with three beds for the take. Moving patients takes a considerable amount of time because all the relatives have to be phoned to say that they are moving; you have to phone up the ward and liaise with the ward staff on the various wards and see what time their beds will be available to move your patients in. We then got a phone call from A & E asking us to take a patient as we are on emergency take and I informed them that they would have to put the patient on hold as we didn't have a bed yet. The three beds that were going to be available on the other end of the ward, the staff nurse was waiting for the HO to finish the rounds so he could come back and write up the TTOs [medication To Take Out] and the doctor's letter, this takes a huge effort on the staff nurse's part to procure and get the HO there to prescribe the TTOs, write the doctor's letter, it can take all day on and off and meanwhile patients are waiting in A & E for a bed that you haven't got.

I then spoke to another social worker about whether a patient would be able to manage at home. I asked if she would come and speak to the patient either today or tomorrow to see what they would need at home, because the wife said that she could no longer manage the husband at home, and I could see where she was coming from. It was then time to do the afternoon drugs [12 noon]. I do think that this new drug policy where the patients have their drugs in their lockers takes twice as long as when we had a drug trolley. Half the time the pharmacy hasn't delivered the drugs to the lockers so you are searching in other people's lockers for the same drug that you know they've got and you know you can use.

The rest of the shift was all right. I then had a look at the student's assessment book with her to see what she wanted to do. Then I did the IVABs [IV antibiotics], made sure the ward was tidy and went into handover. I handed over everything that was said that morning having written it in the Kardex at the desk. We were interrupted several times by various staff: one searching for keys, one to say that the social worker was on the phone, and the pharmacist wanted to talk to me about some TTOs I'd sent down, and some tablets I'd ordered.

You ask me to describe the 8am drug round: I started it at 7.30 and I finished it at 8.10. This was because it takes longer when you are interrupted by doctors. I didn't actually finish the whole round by 8.10, I finished the whole round by about 8.40. But in between time I had been on two doctor's rounds. The doctors normally come on the ward any time between quarter to 8 and 8 o'clock. Mr H and his registrar usually go round before they start operating. You have to have all the dressings down so that they can see the wounds before then. It is not a good idea really because there you are with patients sitting with open wounds with just a clinical sheet over it, while they are expected to have their breakfast and then the domestic starts doing the cleaning! While we went round with the registrar, the orthopaedic doctor came and did a round without a nurse and then walked off the ward. So, when you finish one round, if you haven't been on the other, you then have to bleep them to find out what they said to the patient! One of our consultants is um, quite abusive, verbally, and um loses his temper quite quick and can shout at you on the ward in front of the patients. When they do the rounds, they just give out: 'I want so and so put on this dressing', or 'I want this patient to go home today'. So you pick up a few jobs when they do the rounds. It is very good to take a student round with you especially with Mr H's round. He doesn't like students; he doesn't like staff nurses really! But he doesn't like students more than staff nurses and it's good for them to experience what it is like to be just at the tail end below the HO and what your role is in the doctor's round: basically to be a handmaiden!

We don't always have time to do the students' work things, when you have to go through their book with them and talk to them, and read their work that they have done on your ward, during our shift. Time should be put aside some time during the day, so that you can talk to your students. I feel that the doctors start their rounds too early. I understand why they do this, because obviously they have theatre. But sometimes even if you get out of handover in the morning early, you're still called away from your drug round to go around with the consultant. And sometimes you end up doing two ward rounds, or three ward rounds because you go round with the registrar first, he tells you one thing about a patient, and then the consultant comes round and tells you something totally different. Meanwhile you have already told the patient this is what the registrar has said, because half the time the registrars and the consultants don't speak to the patients, they talk about them at the foot of the bed and the patient doesn't grasp what was said. And then you have to go round and say, 'No, no we're not going to do that now, that was *just* the registrar, the *consultant* says *this*, and this is what we'll do'.

6   The emotional field

Throughout Part I, how emotion is conceptualised has been seen to impact on how emotional labour is understood. This has methodological significance, for emotion is not something that can easily be observed and understood. The methods of data collection and analysis used, therefore, attempt to identify emotion and emotional labour, as the emotions are experienced by, and the emotional labour is carried out by, qualified nursing staff as they occurred in the nursing context. Ward B, an acute vascular and general surgical ward in an English NHS Hospital Trust, forms the context in which this took place. The ward was chosen through expediency. I applied for staffing posts and accepted the first one offered. The nurses agreed to let me work with them and observe their daily routines, which I did for fourteen months; fifteen of them also consented to record audio diaries, and to be interviewed. This chapter explains the methodology and its rationale. It looks at what life was like on Ward B and introduces the nurses who worked there and how this has influenced and informed the research process. It explores how the nurses' stories are retained, while there is also a theoretical analysis exploring the relationship between emotion and emotional labour.

Participant observation

Participant observation was the primary choice of data collection because it was necessary to be inside, or present in, a nursing field in order to situate, observe and understand emotional labour in its context. Fineman (1993: 9) states that 'feelings shape and lubricate social transactions. Feelings contribute to, and reflect, the structure and culture of organisations. Order and control, the very essence of the "organisation" of work, concern what people "do" with their feelings'. Understanding the nature of emotion and emotional labour in the workplace depends on understanding its cultural and structural norms. Identifying and defining the different components of emotion, contrasting and interpreting personal attitudes and displayed emotion in respect to shared feeling rules, can be achieved only from the context of the workplace in which it is carried out. This is because feelings are part of the 'social transactions' carried out in the workplace, thus identifying and understanding them is dependent on the context.

Participant observation also enabled the public display of emotional labour as it occurred within interactive relationships between the labourer and recipient to be observed. This was important because the source of the emotions being managed was more readily identifiable. This process was facilitated because as a member of the ward team, I experienced the everydayness of nursing work and shared similar challenges. I nursed the same patients and worked with the same nurses and health care professionals. I understood the nature of the interaction that took place because I was part of that. Vignette 6, 'An average shift', captures something of what everyday life on Ward B was like. Many of the feelings expressed within it reflect the nature of everyday social transactions that took place. It represents the backdrop behind all the nurses' emotion stories and the context within which their emotional labour was carried out. The participant observation experience helped highlight and interpret the significance of the context to the interaction and helped situate the relationships in which the nurses' emotional labour occurred.

Working with the nurses for over fourteen months meant I developed good relationships with them. This was fundamental to the research because identity and personality are essential to understanding emotion and emotional labour. My role as a staff nurse shaped the relationships I built with the nurses, and subsequently, how I interpreted the data. 'Role . . . might be appropriately defined as processual and ever changing and subject to negotiation over and over again' (de Laine 2000: 95). At the beginning orientation towards the ward and to vascular surgical nursing shaped the initial experiences. All new nurses are allocated a preceptor to assist in this process (preceptors oversee and assess their competency, professional development and adjustment to the ward). However, within eight months I was a preceptor myself to a newly qualified nurse Susan (Vignette 4, 'The murderer'). Successfully fulfilling the role of staff nurse was vital because peer status is important in developing a rapport and establishing relationships based on trust and respect; role performance is important in establishing peer status. Being efficient and competent in my nursing care was essential to establishing trust, and building up relationships with the other nurses. Vignette 6 illustrates how busy the nurses on Ward B were. Ensuring the safety and wellbeing of the patients and fulfilling the role of staff nurse properly were of primary importance. Thus, as an active participant, the degree of observation carried out was also limited.

In addition, while it was possible to observe emotions as they were expressed spontaneously, it was not always possible to identify those that were being managed. For the very management process involves suppressing one's own emotions for the benefit of others. Suppressed emotions are not visible emotions. Participant observation alone does not allow for a deep understanding of people's personal and private emotions, or allow for how this might contrast with their public expression. However, establishing relationships with the nurses as a result of the participant observation was important to the depth of their confidences in their audio diary and interviews. Observing the nurses during the participant observation also meant that the beginning of their emotion trajectory, as it relates to the inner dialogue, could be identified and followed up through their diaries.

Audio diaries

In Archer's (2000) work, emotions were seen as personal commentaries on the things that concern individuals because they inform, and then are transformed, through the inner dialogue over a period of time. In order to access more private expressions of emotion and to track their trajectory audio diaries were used. An advantage of diaries is that respondents tend to use them to vent their feelings (Morrison and Galloway 1996). They were useful therefore because they encouraged the nurses to express those more private and personal feelings that they kept hidden from public view. Because these were their personal feelings, they were more closely tied to their sense of personal identity and often reflected their inner dialogue, as evident in Vignette 5, 'Maxine's rant'. To encourage this, the nurses were asked to describe how they were feeling after the shift they had just done and why in their diary.

A further advantage of diaries is that they represent 'I am here and it is exactly now; a diary is a document for the now; a particular moment in time' (Plummer 2001: 48). Audio diaries were used because at the end of a shift, especially a fourteen and a half-hour one, it is quicker and easier to spend ten minutes talking into a Dictaphone than half an hour writing it down. In addition, several of the nurses were non-native English speakers and might have been deterred from participating due to written language difficulties. The spoken word also portrayed a sense of the immediacy of their feelings (Plummer 2001). The 'here and now' was captured through their verbal communication, their intonation, emphasis, tone of voice and speed of their words, conveying their emotion much more readily than if they had written them.

The audio diaries, therefore, captured the spontaneous, immediate nature of emotion conveyed through the verbal expression of the person experiencing it, complementing what was observed in the participant observation. Plummer also comments on how diaries can extend beyond the here and now, slowly building up a more representative picture of the individual's life experience. 'Diaries are certainly valuable in talking to the subjectivity of a particular moment; but they usually will go beyond this to a conception of some whole' (Plummer 2001: 49). Although the nurses kept their audio diaries for an average of only four to six weeks, a picture of their individual emotion trajectories was built up. This was assisted by the relationships built with the nurses, both prior to, and after, the diaries were completed.

The diaries represented aspects of life on Ward B from February to October 2001 when the final diary was completed. In that time, some nurses left, and new ones arrived; sometimes the ward was frenetically busy, at other times calmer. Some nurses worked seven and a half-hour shifts, others fourteen hours; some nurses did their diaries on night duty. This resulted in patterns of emotion response and expression and their possible causes being illustrated irrespective of individual emotion response, while a more in-depth individual insight was gained. Shared and individual insight can be seen in Vignette 6. What I 'hear' when I read Paula's account, for example, is the voice of a mature and experienced nurse – similar to that of the other senior nurses. She gives the appearance of being placid, taking everything in her stride as she meets it. This is represented in her tone and in the pace of her voice, which is very measured. Paula was also particularly good with student nurses, who used to gravitate towards her – also evident in her narrative. Underneath this, however, is a strand of cynicism which emerges when she talks about the doctors. Here her tone becomes sarcastic. This is a characteristic individual to Paula. She was not fond of the doctors. She also felt that the NHS took advantage of nurses, working them until they had little left to give. This attitude comes through in her comment about working in her own time to meet her students' learning needs.

The diaries were also effective in tracking the 'trajectory' of the nurses (de Laine 2000), and offered a 'running account' and 'description of their activities, experiences and feelings' (Henerson *et al.* 1987: 29). Diaries have been used to explore the working lives of people who have very little time and are hard to follow due to the fragmentary nature and the quantity of the work they do (Morrison and Galloway 1996). The diaries were used therefore to observe the nurses through their own eyes, complementing the participant observation.

To facilitate this, the nurses were given diary format sheets, which guided their observations. These were based on six everyday routine nursing responsibilities reflecting a typical day's trajectory: handover, the doctor's ward rounds, the drugs round, wound care and clinical skills, mentoring students and discharge planning. They were asked to describe what had occurred during the 8 o'clock drug round, what time they started and finished the round, did anything happen to interrupt it, did they have everything they required for it, and how did they feel about the whole process and why? Vignette 6 illustrates how this worked. These routines were also selected because they could be controversial. This is highlighted in Vignette 6, when Paula mentions the 8am drugs round and the doctor's rounds. These were contentious because they occurred at similar times. Mentoring students also created conflict because they required constant supervision and the nurses were also expected to teach and assess their skills. There were often more students per shift than staff nurses, which provoked anger and resentment about the extra workload involved in looking after them. Through the diaries these attitudes were captured, augmenting what was observed in the participant observation.

The diaries linked with the participant observation because the nurses told their stories to me. For example, Paula says, 'You ask me to describe the 8 o'clock drug round'. The relationships that I had with the nurses were integral to the diaries. In telling their stories they would also be imagining my response to them. Thus in Vignette 5, as Maxine tells her story she is appealing to my understanding about what has happened and how she feels when she splutters 'you know; you know . . . !'. It was also possible that the nurses may be describing events in which I had been present, or patients whom I knew. For example, in Vignette 2 Amelia says about Alix, 'You know what he is like . . .' The audio diaries were successful because they related directly to life on Ward B while also reflecting the inner life of the nurse. Connecting the two was my individual relationship with each nurse.

Interviews

This relationship was continued in the interviews. The interviews offered an opportunity to discuss the emotions expressed in the diaries, several months later – allowing for the passage of time. Before conducting the interviews, the audio diaries were transcribed so that questions could be asked about the emotions expressed in them. Each interview was personalised to facilitate a fuller explanation of the events provoking the feelings expressed in the diaries and in order to give the nurses an opportunity to interpret them. In discussing the events and feelings recorded in the diaries, the nurses were asked how they were feeling about these events at the time of the interview in order to contrast their feelings with those expressed on the audio diary. For example, if the nurse had expressed anger or frustration in the diary, in the interview her attention was drawn to that section of the transcript, and she was invited to describe her feelings and the event that elicited them more fully. Then she would be asked to comment on how it made her feel now in comparison to then. The interviews were used therefore to complete the trajectory begun in the participant observation and the audio diaries.

As Archer (2000) notes, emotions reflect issues in which individuals invest themselves. Identifying the individual values, beliefs and attitudes of the nurses that they had invested themselves in, was important in establishing which emotions mattered, and how this reflected their individuality in respect to shared feeling rules, values, beliefs, norms and attitudes. Thus, the interviews also included structured questions in order to establish their individual responses to them. The relevance of this can be seen in Vignette 1 'Half measures', where Paris identifies what aspects of nursing care are important to her. Other questions asked why they had decided to become a nurse, what they most enjoyed and disliked about it and whether they had ever thought of leaving and if so why? In addition, the interview built up a wider picture of the individual nurse's family background and social circumstances. As Archer (2000) notes, our family and social lives can influence our motivation, attitudes and values in our working lives. Pertinent questions about the structure and organisation of the ward were also asked in order to encourage the nurses to express their opinions and satisfactions about the difficulties and problems in nursing.

The purpose of the interviews was threefold. First, they aimed to produce narrative accounts about individual nurses in which to set the context of their emotional nursing lives. Second, they were conducted as an interactive dialogue between nurse and interviewer in which various situations at work were discussed and interpreted that reflected their feelings, opinions and attitudes about them. Third, they aimed to follow through the emotion trajectories started in the audio diaries.

During the interviews the nurses were asked about their personal and private emotions and the difference between their private and public personas. Establishing a rapport between interviewer and interviewee is seen as essential to successful interviewing. Interviews should be seen as collaborative ventures that cannot take place if trust and respect between interviewer and interviewee is missing because the interviewee is essentially giving a personal account of themselves (Kikumura 1998). However, because the relationships developed with the nurses occurred over an extensive period of time, in which many experiences were shared, the relationship went far beyond a general 'rapport'. Minister (1991: 34) claims that overall, women support one another by 'defining themselves in terms of their roles and relationships to others'. Understanding one's relationship in respect to others contributes towards the position held in the group, and impacts on the kind and nature of the relationships built within the field, affecting personal feelings towards individuals and the group as a whole (Prus 1996). This was particularly relevant because it was the nurses' emotions that were sought in the diaries and the interviews. What the nurses shared about their emotions and how they interpreted them with me, and how I analysed them therefore, was rooted in the dynamic relationship between me and the nurse. To understand this more fully it is necessary to understand life on Ward B and the dynamics between the staff. For as Tonkin (1992: 97) asserts 'narratives [should] be seen as social actions situated in particular times and places and directed by individual tellers to specific audiences'.

Ward B

Ward B was sometimes an uncomfortable place to work. Before the participant observation began, the previous G grade sister had been arrested and subsequently convicted of unprofessional conduct. Daisy, the new ward sister, had been in post for only a couple of months. The sheer quantity and pace of the work combined with too few human resources made optimum care hard to achieve, generating stress and tension. The distribution of the workload was therefore extremely significant. The nurses were divided into two teams: A and B, and C, D and E, matching the geographical layout of the ward (see Figure 6.1): A and B team looked after A and B bay and side rooms 4, 5 and 6, whereas C, D and E team looked after C, D and E bay and side rooms 1, 2 and 3. There were not enough qualified nurses to ensure that a nurse from each team was on duty every shift, but the aim of the duty roster was to ensure that a minimum of two staff nurses were on duty per shift, one for each team. It was possible, therefore, that on some shifts only D grades would be on duty. Thus, D grades were expected to undertake the same nursing responsibilities as E or F grades. HCAs were allocated in a similar way. Their responsibilities included carrying out the majority of patient hygiene, dressing and nutritional care, bed making, simple toileting needs, basic observations and some dressings, overseen by the nurses.

Because the work demand was greater than the human and material resources available to meet it, and because there was a flattening of the official hierarchy, there was no clear chain of command. The nurses on Ward B were organised into unofficial but clearly defined cliques. Each clique had its own identity, social norms, attitudes, values and feeling rules. Most of the nurses denied being in a clique, but each one had her place.

> **Maxine:** The ward is getting worse. You are getting your little cliques. And there are two sets of them. And I'm not; I will not get in a clique for love nor money. I have my friends, I have two friends from the ward, but I wouldn't call us a clique and I wouldn't make people uncomfortable if we were on together. I never say that we have to go to break together and leave the ward uncovered, because it just doesn't happen. I'd hate to think that I'd make anybody feel uncomfortable if one of my friends was on.

The impact of the cliques on the ward should not be underestimated. The divisions and jostling for place between the cliques was linked to patterns of bullying, which were habitual and passed down, with some of the nurses, previously victims of the bullies, becoming perpetrators themselves. Working with members of a different clique could be traumatic, whereas working with friends could be enjoyable, regardless of how busy the shift was. Thus, everybody belonged to a clique in order to both identify with some colleagues and protect themselves from others.

> **Kate:** I was going into work and I was uptight, and I would get into work, and they would be there, and I would be on edge and I'd be watching myself all the time, watching what I said. I wouldn't converse with anybody. I wouldn't even converse with any of them about what I had done the night before. They didn't know anything about me you know. And it was only when I was working with people that I knew really well, that it was nice shifts that I opened up. And I could feel

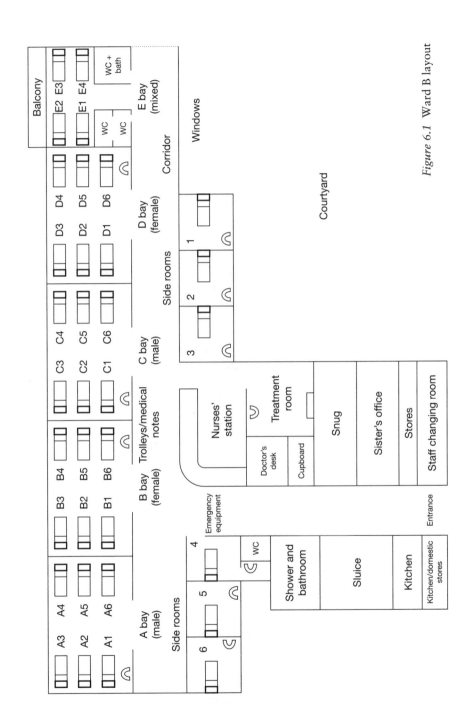

Figure 6.1 Ward B layout

myself relaxing, and I didn't know how relaxed I was with these people until I realised how uptight I was with the crowd of people I didn't want to be with.

The cliques were divided into two alpha groups, which I have named the 'seniors' and the 'populars', and the beta group. The *alpha seniors* were the longest standing nurses, married or divorced with teenage or grown-up children, and had been nursing for at least ten years. They were mostly E grades. The members of this clique considered themselves to be above ward politics. They were the most knowledgeable and experienced nurses on the ward, characterised by pragmatic attitudes, and unafraid of hard work. They saw themselves as professional people and were quietly confident about their nursing abilities. The seniors were a group who seldom expressed their feelings. Thus, it was surprising to discover how resentful they were about Ward B and how cynical they were about nursing generally, in their diaries and interviews. On the whole, the alpha seniors tacitly colluded with the bullying rather than perpetrating it. They did this by participating in group status conflict, accepting the actions of the bullies and ignoring the consequences to the bullied. They considered that they lacked power and seldom asserted any authority. This was partly because when the senior sister, Daisy, joined the ward, she became a member of the populars, making them an alpha group. This resulted in much jostling between the two, and increased the resentment felt by the alpha seniors.

The *alpha populars*, a mix of Ds and Es, were much younger. They were outgoing and very sociable, often going out after work together. They liked to have a laugh on the ward. The populars were responsible for the majority of the bullying and thought that ward politics were very important. In contrast to the seniors, they acted as if they had a great deal of power. The G grade, Daisy, was only 37 years old, and was a natural member of the popular group. She enjoyed having a laugh and going out with her friends.

> **Daisy:** I think I've got a nice personality, I think I'm quite a good leader, I'm always having a laugh and a joke. When I first went to that ward, they hadn't heard anyone laugh for months, you know, and the patients do like it. I always remember one Sunday morning when I went in, right let's get the radio on, Steve Wright love songs and the women absolutely loved it and the patients were going to the other nurses 'that sister is so nice because she has a laugh, she has a joke, she does this, she does that'.

Daisy wanted to be liked, and being liked and being popular became a ward value, supported by feeling rules that defined the popular group. Within the popular group, therefore, individuals who were liked and considered sociable and outgoing were similarly considered to be good nurses. They were commended for how friendly they were to each other, irrespective of their nursing abilities.

Daisy: Whether we like it or not, there is this sort of tribal stuff going on, wherever we work, it's all tribal. The job I am in, I've got to be politically correct with everybody. You know. But good luck to Kate 'cos you need people like her to say 'Why are you doing it like that [being outspoken]?' But I wouldn't. I like to be liked I wouldn't want to be not spoken to, or to upset people. I hate the idea of thinking that I'd upset somebody, you know?

The majority of the nurses in the ***beta group*** were culturally different from the other nurses due to their ethnicity, race or religion. These nurses were regularly bullied. New nurses went into the beta group by default; they could, however, graduate into the seniors or the populars. Beta group nurses identified with one another as the objects of prejudice, and from shared feelings of inadequacy due to bullying. They were characterised by their desire to support one another and demonstrated strong feelings of empathy for anybody seen to be struggling on the ward. They often had little confidence in their own nursing abilities. Paris, the F grade sister, was in the beta group due to her ethnicity. However, she was well respected by everyone and was seldom the object of the bullying.

The HCAs were also affiliated to the different subgroups. The longest standing HCAs typically associated with the alpha seniors, the younger ones with the alpha populars and those who were ethnically or racially different with the beta group. The jockeying for power between the RGNs, however, also provided the HCAs with leverage, so their groupings were not as fixed as the staff nurses' were. For example, a HCA who was nominally associated with the alpha seniors, but who wanted to go for a cigarette break, might obtain permission from an alpha popular when denied by an alpha senior. HCAs also have a great deal of power because they undertake the majority of basic hands-on nursing care. However, it is the staff nurse who is accountable for that care, provoking conflict.

Maria: They [HCAs] have got so much to say all the time! They are not doing a nurse's job but they are interfering all the time. At work everybody should know their place what to do. If somebody wants to be nurse, then why doesn't she finish training? I hear their opinions, 'No I don't want to be in charge, it is very stressful', but when she is not doing what I ask her she is complaining or something, you know, or interfering or changing my decision, if she doesn't agree then it should be different way. When I ask them, 'Would you like to be a nurse?' they say 'No, never. It is too stressful, too much responsibility'. 'Then why are you interfering? Why are you challenging my opinion now?'

The allocation of work was the means by which alpha nurses could establish primacy and isolate lower status nurses. At the beginning of a shift, whoever was 'top dog' at the time allocated the staff to one of the teams. C, D and E were always allocated two staff nurses and two HCAs if staffing levels allowed. A and B, on the other hand, was allocated one staff nurse and two HCAs. This effectively isolated the staff nurse working in A and B. Thus, allocating to A and B was the primary means of establishing primacy on the ward. Vignette 5 'Maxine's rant' demonstrates the effectiveness of this strategy. The nurse allocated to A and B was usually in the beta group. If none of the nurses on duty was in the beta group, then the alpha group with the most nurses on duty took C, D and E bay, isolating the nurse from the other alpha group in A and B. Further alienation was achieved by allocating the least experienced or agency HCAs to A and B, while the most experienced HCAs worked in C, D and E.

The division of labour between the teams and within C, D and E was also uneven. Both C (male) and B (female) bay were high dependency bays; the only difference between the two was the gender of the patients. C bay, for no discernible reason, was considered more specialised than B bay. This belief resulted in C bay (plus one side room) being allocated one nurse to it, whereas the nurse in B bay also had to look after A bay and three other side rooms. Because the nurse in C bay only had seven patients, the other staff nurse in D and E had to look after twelve. Although the majority of these were usually low dependency patients, the workload was still high due to the number of discharges, admissions and theatre cases in these bays. Owing to the myth that the high dependency patients in C bay needed a more experienced nurse, an E grade nearly always looked after C bay. In the fourteen months I was on Ward B, I worked in C bay three times. It took me nearly six months to realise that C bay was no more specialised than B bay. The C bay myth conceals the truth that control of C bay establishes the pecking order for the day. The nurse in C bay gives the impression that she is calm and efficient, easily accomplishing her workload in comparison to everyone else. In doing so, she establishes her superiority. This status then gives her the right to express disgust, irritation and frustration at the other nurses who are rushing around, finding the accomplishment of their entire workload more difficult. Looking after seven patients, however, is simply easier than fifteen or twelve.

> **Maria:** I will tell you what I like to do is C bay because I can concentrate you know. I can have all C bay poorly patients. You can concentrate on your patients, every time you are going in; you can see all the poorly patients together. Yes. So, I prefer to work in C, D and E and do C bay. And I am not surprised that some of staff they are very keen to do C bay, even though you have got very poorly patients, because you are concentrating in one bay, you don't have to go to D, E, you know you don't bother with what is going on there. You have got only one bay and if you go to C1 [bed number] you can still see the others. If you are checking urine output you are checking everybody all together. Yes. Yes

you can check bum properly you can apply cream, you can change TED stockings [special surgical stockings], stupid things, but nursing you know, it's nursing. You can check IV fluids in time, everything yes. And anyway it is only six patients, so you can remember whose urine output is okay, whose is not, who has got PCA [patient controlled analgesia] or epidural. Sometimes if you have got all A and B you have got people all over, it is confusing and you can mix patients. It is very dangerous as well from this point of view. Sometimes I wasn't sure who has drain, whether it is Redivac, or Robinson's, I couldn't remember, or remind myself because I didn't wash the patients, and if I didn't look after everybody in A bay, I was concentrating on B bay or something you know. I didn't know if it was epidural or morphine, I had to go and check. We are only human beings we can't be everywhere and remember everything. Yes. It is better for us, it is only six people, so you can look after them proper and you can remember and you can see them all the time you know.

An important feeling rule on Ward B was concerned with how much work was achieved irrespective of the demand in relation to the resources. A good shift was defined by how much was accomplished, and a bad shift, the opposite. Feelings of satisfaction and/or dissatisfaction, pride or shame were measured according to this rule and nurses were expected to recognise and express guilt if they did not achieve the maximum workload possible.

Kay: A bad shift would be a very busy one that I got nothing done in. Huh! (*Laughs*) Things that I wanted to do but couldn't do. Not busy from the workload really, I don't shy away from hard work. I will work as hard as everybody else does. It's when you have so many things you have to do, and you can't because there just isn't any time. If you didn't have any breaks, or you didn't have your five minute breather or a visit to the loo . . . it still wouldn't get it all done. That's a bad shift.

Catherine: What would you say a good shift is?

The exact opposite, because even if it's busy, you get everything done that you set out to do, or at least started. Like in the case of a discharge plan, in that you have done the first stage. Yes, it is very unsatisfactory to not be able to finish something, or to not start something that you know should have been started. I have had shifts when I have gone from a late to an early, when I haven't had time to do anything on the late and I've said when I have handed over to the night staff that I haven't had time to do this, but I'll do it in the morning. Usually it's not too drastic a thing um, and I don't feel too guilty about it because sometimes it's been, when it's been really wild right up until report and I really just haven't had the chance, but it's very, very unsatisfactory to do that. And sometimes the night staff will do it if they can, if they've got help. No, a good shift is when you can do all of that and go off knowing that you have done it all.

The C bay myth supports a Ward B value that the quantity of work accomplished per shift separates good efficient nurses from bad, less efficient nurses. Thus, the nurse in C bay who successfully manages all her workload not only gains status rights, but also holds moral superiority over those who find this more difficult. Clark (1990) notes that emotion can be used as 'place markers' in establishing status where social place is relative. These are what she terms 'the ploys of emotional micropolitics' (Clark 1990: 305). The bullying tactics used on Ward B were designed to lower the self-esteem of some nurses in the eyes of others by shaming them and lowering their status while elevating their own. By controlling the allocation of work, the bullies could ensure that the least number of HCAs and the largest number of students were given to the nurse in A and B. The other nurses would then question her competency and closely observe and monitor her work, expressing distrust at her decisions. Placing her performance under intense scrutiny makes the nurse appear incompetent and unable to sustain her workload. When the bullied nurse subsequently failed to complete all of her tasks, the other nurses could then express anger at her failure and draw attention to it by resentfully completing it herself, or allocating 'extra' support to that team, thereby depriving the other team. This strategy was employed against Maxine in Vignette 6. Hopfl and Linstead (1993: 77) suggest that the consequence of such tactics is that 'the burden of sustaining consistency becomes too great for the actor to bear', lowering the bullied nurses' sense of self-esteem and resulting in a low status place among the nurses, while those who have induced this are elevated.

> **Maria:** I was scared. I noticed that everybody checked on me all the time, whether I know my job or not. They observed me and was checking me, not just the nursing bits but the health care bits as well. For example am I coping with drugs or with washes? Actually, I don't like people observing me, even visitors. I like to be if I am taking clips out or drains or pumps or something you know, I prefer to be on my own. It wasn't just staff nurses it was the health care assistants as well. They make me feel stupid.

As a new nurse and a researcher, I was allocated to the beta group and initially experienced much of the bullying. These experiences influenced the relationships I formed with the staff. I developed strong relationships based on empathy and respect with those nurses who were also bullied. With the bullies themselves, dislike hindered the development of any kind of constructive relationship to begin with; initially it was hard to respect those who were in a position to act, but did not. Hearing about how the bullying was affecting others in the audio diaries and listening to others openly judge their colleagues was often difficult. However, all the nurses showed me trust and respect in their willingness to participate in the research, and in the degree to which they openly reflected about their personal feelings and opinions in their diaries and interviews. In the interviews, therefore, either the level of trust and empathy was very high due to shared experience, or a re-evaluation of the relationship between me and the other nurse occurred.

Because of the undercurrent of bullying and the pace and quantity of work, Ward B was not always the most comfortable environment in which to work. Despite this, the staff always aimed to provide the best care possible for their patients. When emergencies happened or the patients were going through particularly difficult times, the nurses worked together putting their patients' needs first. Ward B was an emotional field: appreciating these dynamics is fundamental to understanding the interaction between the nurses, and to identifying, interpreting and analysing the nurses' emotions and emotional labour.

Analysing the data

Three tools of analysis were developed in order to identify emotion as fully as possible and consider its relationship with emotional labour in the context in which they occurred, maintain the integrity and emotionality of the nurses' stories while extracting theoretical relevance from them, and minimise any bias I had towards the nurses, without losing the value that my relationship with them brought to the analysis. These tools were:

- narrative
- reflexivity and transference
- theoretical frameworks: Hochschild's notion of emotion management, feeling rules, surface and deep acting; Archer's emotion orders and inner dialogue.

Narrative

Narratives are told as stories. The benefits of these are that as the nurses' stories unfold, they convey their feelings and emotions within the boundaries of their experiences at work. Essentially they are 'emotional communiqués' (Sandelands and Boudens 2000: 58) which, in the expression of their emotion, illustrate the nurses' understanding of social norms and values in their actions, and in their explanation of the behaviour of others. The nurses' narratives are represented throughout the book, encapsulated in vignettes preceding every chapter. The nurses' stories in all the vignettes clearly 'communicate the life and feeling of work' (Sandelands and Boudens 2000: 58), and they invite us to share that with them. An advantage of this is that the reader can engage with the nurses' experiences

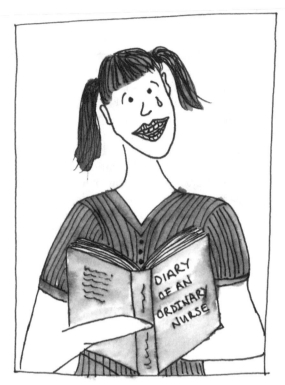

'Nursing stories'

before interpretation is suggested in the chapter that follows. In addition, the dynamic structure described above is revealed within the stories the nurses tell of life on Ward B. In Part I, their emotions, feeling rules, attitudes and values represented in the vignettes are refracted through a theoretical lens. In Part II, the vignettes are analysed in depth. The narrative format forms part of that process.

Stories are used by people in the workplace to share and define feelings experienced in groups and to help individuals understand where they fit in relation to others.

> By representing feeling at work, stories serve two important functions in the workplace. One is to collect and communicate the life and feeling of work. With stories people can grab hold of feelings that would be otherwise inexpressible and unmemorable. For better or worse, stories reinforce and amplify feelings at work. A second and probably more important function of stories is to define the group for those inside and outside the group. By virtue of who is included in them and who they are told to, stories are almost implicitly about an 'us' and a 'them'.

Stories are thus a powerful way that people learn about who they are and who they like and dislike.

(Sandelands and Boudens 2000: 58)

Narratives have four elements: 'boundaries, dynamic tensions, growth (movement) and possibility' which can help shape the process of analysis. First, 'boundaries distinguish a story from other elements in the flow of communication. Boundaries allow a listener to appreciate the story openly for what it is' (Sandelands and Boudens 2000: 57). The vignettes represent large extracts from the nurses' diaries and interviews. These narratives are mostly unedited so that the individual nurse's voice comes through without interpretation and analysis. Boundaries are also important because the context, characters and purpose of the story are defined within them, marking out the parameters within which analysis takes place. Second, 'the story's dynamic tensions capture the listener's interest and draw him or her into the story by eliciting curiosity about what will happen next and especially about whether everything will turn out all right' (Sandelands and Boudens 2000: 57). Emotions are felt, experienced and expressed; they make things real to us. The difficulty with grappling with theory and demonstrating logical pathways and connections in academic writing is that the experience of embodied emotion becomes lost. In the dynamic tensions within a story, however, the reader is drawn in, identifying with the needs, feelings and concerns of the individual in the story. It also means that emotions can be more readily recognised within the text as the purpose of the story is to share them. Thus, even when theory is used to help identify the emotions, those emotions should be recognisable from within the story. Third,

> growth is that element of the story which projects a pathway for tensions to be elaborated and eventually released. Growth is a significant element of the story because it affirms life in the dimension of time. All living things change over time and most change in ways that indicate a cumulative development.
>
> (Sandelands and Boudens 2000: 57)

The combination of participant observation, audio diaries and interviews was designed to enable the significance of time to emotion and emotional labour to be captured. The use of narrative helps illustrate that time flow. In addition, as individuals grow and develop, their inner dialogue emerges through the trajectory of their narratives. In some of the vignettes, excerpts from the audio diaries and interviews have been combined where they specifically relate to each other. In others, chronological entries from the diary are shown. In this way 'a pathway for tensions to be elaborated and eventually released' as they emerge within the nurse's narrative are captured. Fourth, 'possibility appears in most artistic stories as a hint or an indication that while a reconciliation of the story's immediate tensions may have been reached, there are questions and unresolved issues to ponder' (Sandelands and Boudens 2000: 57). The realm of possibility creates a space within the story for interpretation and anticipation of its significance and potential resolution. Within this space, theoretical understandings about the relationship between emotion and emotional labour are extracted from the stories. Together these components of the narrative 'establish a semblance of life and feeling' in a snapshot all can participate in.

Reflexivity and transference

Letting the stories stand alone, however, does not enable understanding about the significance of emotion to emotional labour and the impact of emotional labour on nursing care. The vignettes, drawn from the audio diaries, interviews and participant observation are not works of fiction. To develop some degree of intersubjective coherence between theory and method without losing the reality of the emotion experience represented in the stories, sociological reflexivity was also used in the process of analysis.

In his commentary on the study of human lived experience, Prus (1996) considers how reflexivity (which he terms reflectivity) can help achieve this.

> Human group life is reflective. Through interaction with others and by taking the viewpoint of the other with respect to oneself, people develop capacities to become objects of their own awareness. By attending to the viewpoint of 'the other' (what Mead [1934] terms 'role taking'), people are able to attribute meanings to their own 'essences' and to develop lines of action that take themselves (and other objects) into account . . . Reflectivity is not only a product of ongoing association, but assumes its significance as 'human agency' when people go about their activities.
>
> (Prus 1996: 15–16)

The advantage of reflexivity is that it allows the researcher to take the 'viewpoint of the other with respect to oneself' (Prus 1996: 15) allowing meaning to be drawn from the experiences, relationships and data gained from the field without the research objective being lost. It also extends the process of analysis as a continuation of those experiences and relationships. In effect the dual roles of researcher-nurse and nurse-colleague become more explicit within the analysis process. As researcher-nurse I entered the field and recorded my observations in order to identify the social norms, values, attitudes, feeling rules, and the skills, practices and emotional labour of the nurses in the negotiation and renegotiation of daily nursing life. From this the boundaries of each narrative are identified by interpreting the context, and explaining the situations and interactions being recounted. In this sense as researcher-nurse I become the narrator of their story, building up a picture that represents the dynamic tensions and growth and development of their emotional representations and daily activities. This kind of reflexivity objectifies the relationships developed in the field, as information, interpretation and analysis are drawn from them. Jacoby (1984), drawing on Martin Buber (1922), calls this the 'I-It' attitude.

> The 'I-It' attitude would mean that the world and one's fellow men [*sic*] are seen only as objects. This can of course take place on many different levels. People can be objects of my reflections and my criticisms, but I can also turn them into objects of my own needs and my own fears, which means that other people get used for one's own conscious and very often unconscious purposes. The boss of a big company might for instance use his staff as objects that he needs for the financial growth of his firm, considering people only from the point of their usefulness. I-It relationships can also be for mutual benefit.
>
> (Jacoby 1984: 62)

At the beginning of any social research project this is the kind of relationship the researcher has with the research subject. Negotiating access often revolves around the mutual benefit of the relationship. In choosing which excerpts from the nurses' diaries and interviews to include in the analysis as researcher-nurse, those experiences and relationships are turned into objects for the purposes of the research. Sustaining an I-It relationship with the nurses is a necessary part of the reflexive process both in understanding emotion and in retaining the researcher's voice in the text. Assuming the role of researcher-nurse achieves a degree of objectivity in observation and analysis and in understanding emotion from this perspective, by separating the self from the others. An essential component of this process is the application of the theoretical concepts and frameworks discussed in Part I of the book. This form of reflexivity can also be extended to interpret the 'I-It' attitude between the nurses. This can help untangle the dynamics in their relationships without my subjective interpretation overdominating.

The value and necessity of the relationships formed with the nurses is brought to the reflexive analysis process in the role of nurse-colleague. While it is possible to observe emotion expression and exchange, to understand it without relating to the real life otherness of the people experiencing it is to miss the import of the emotion. Understanding the emotional representation of the nurses is also self-reflective because it represents my individual experiences of how I felt about the situation and how I imagined the others felt, in my role as nurse-colleague; through this, I take on their viewpoint in respect to myself. However, as Prus (1996) observes:

> people do not associate with one another in random or undifferentiated manners but tend to develop more particularistic bonds or affiliations with other members of the communities in which they find themselves. This premise not only acknowledges the differing identities (i.e., self and other definitions) that people attach to one another, but is also mindful

of the loyalties, disaffections, and other interactional styles that emerge between people in the course of human interaction.

(Prus 1996: 16)

This can be considered problematic in analysis because it is too subjective. However, the relationships formed with the nurses, and their representations of those relationships with me and with others, whether accurate or not, draws a picture of how emotion operates, representing its interactive relational nature. It cannot be taken out of the analysis because it represents my relationship with them as a colleague encapsulated within the audio diaries and the interviews. Thus, their self-reflexivity and mine as individuals and members of the group enabled 'the standpoint of the other to "converse with themselves about themselves"' (Prus 1996: 16). In the process, meaning about themselves, me and the others in their role as nurses and in the activities spoken about was reflected on. Jacoby (1984) refers to this as the 'I-Thou' attitude:

> The 'I-Thou' attitude would involve a relation to the genuine otherness of the other person. It would mean that I in my own totality am relating to Thou in his or her own totality. Consciously I may have the attitude of letting the other person live in his own right and not making an object of him for my own purposes. But how do I know this does not happen unconsciously all the same? I have to be fairly well aware of my own width and length, of my own needs, fantasies and value standards, otherwise they will get projected onto the other person who automatically becomes partly an object of my own. To relate to the otherness of Thou, I have to know who I am. Psychologically speaking it would involve . . . recognising what belongs to me and what belongs to the other person.
>
> (Jacoby 1984: 63)

Understanding the difference between I-It and I-Thou is essential to identifying the import of emotion in social processes because it involves either the elicitation of empathy or the absence of empathy towards another. Empathy is being able to relate to another person, to consider their point of view in relation to oneself and is the first step in holding a relationship that represents something of one person to another and vice versa. Without a degree of empathy, attempting to analyse emotions of others would be meaningless. This kind of analysis is extended to all the nurses, but most particularly to Kate, a nurse with whom I had a high degree of empathy. Extracts are predominantly taken from her diary and interview in the following analysis chapters. This enables a more consistent analysis of the emergence and importance of personal identity in emotion processes, which the reader can also engage with by coming to know one individual more fully.

An advantage of reflexivity is that it 'is not only a product of ongoing association, but it assumes significance as "human agency" when people go about their activities' (Prus 1996: 17). Reflexivity 'is dialectically experienced and expressed as people engage in instances of definition, interpretation, intentionality, assessment and minded activities over time' (Prus 1996: 17). Thus reflexivity arises from the interactive relationship between the researcher and the research participants. As discussed in Chapter 4, unconscious emotions can also emerge from interactive encounters. Bion (1979) suggests that 'when two characters or personalities meet, an emotional storm is created. If they make a sufficient contact to be aware of each other, an emotional state is produced by the conjunction of these two individuals' (cited in Symington 1986: 29). Such an understanding requires a degree of awareness of one's own and the other person's personality in order to reflexively discern what those emotions are (Jacoby 1984). This reflexive awareness is where the unconscious nature of emotion resides in an identifiable way. Although it is unconscious emotion, it is still part of that 'dialectically experienced and expressed' social relationship. For between people, emotion states collide, impacting, bouncing and feeding off one another, creating a further emotional state born out of that interaction. The way in which this occurs is known as *transference*: a psychoanalytic term. 'Transference', Craib explains,

> involves projection, and is the fundamental way in which all human relationships, from before birth onwards are formed. We imagine what our parents are thinking and feeling, and later in life what our partners and friends are thinking and feeling and what our children will be, or are thinking and feeling; we are all born into our parents' phantasies. There is a sense in which a human relationship, any human relationship, involves an exchange of parts . . . and it follows that any relationship will involve some degree of transference.
>
> (Craib 2001: 196)

Transference is a necessary process through which individuals see reflections of themselves in others, thereby creating a sense of self-identity in their own estimation and in others'. This is similar to Cooley's (1922) notion of the 'Looking Glass Self'. Transference is also essential to how relationships are formed and perceived. Jacoby claims that

> every human relationship is coloured to a certain degree by transference, that is, by unconscious projections. Our relationships have to be fitted into our own 'world design'. The more conscious we are of ourselves, the more we can relate to the otherness of another person.
>
> (Jacoby 1984: 70)

Transference is therefore an inherently interactive and relational encounter (even in phantasy an 'other' is involved). Transference is used here as a tool to uncover unconscious emotion revealed through a reflexive analysis of how the nurse relates to 'the otherness' of the other nurses she describes in her story.

Freud (1915b, 1925), who first developed the concept, suggests that transference involves the patient *projecting* feelings of affection and security that stem from others in their life (such as the infantile love expectation of their parents) onto the therapist, falling in love with them. In fact, Freud believed that unless a patient could achieve transference, they would not respond to psychotherapy (Jacoby 1984; Joseph 1989; Craib 1998). Klein (1997 [1955]) developed the notion of transference to include the projection and enactment of many emotional fragments of past relationships, beyond that of love (Spilius 1988; Craib 2001). She suggests that transference involves *projective identification* where one person unconsciously gets rid of parts of the self, including destructive emotions like anger and hate as well as love, into others. *Introjective identification*, on the other hand, is where the other person unconsciously takes those unwanted attributes projected by the other person into themselves and then acts them out. For Klein, this process of transference is related to the paranoid-schizoid position, where the ego from infancy has learned to split the loved object from the hated object. Klein considers this splitting to be necessary for distinguishing between core experiences of love and hate, and therefore in facilitating a healthy emotional life. This process of projection and introjection is considered to occur in the total transference situation between a patient and their analyst (Joseph 1989). 'I-It' and 'I-Thou' reflexivity requires an unconscious and conscious awareness of self in respect to other: Jacoby (1984) notes that this involves processes of transference. An attempt is made therefore to discern aspects of projection and introjection in the way the nurses describe the otherness of their colleagues by examining their 'I-It' and 'I-Thou' attitudes. Through this, fragments of unconscious emotion are made more visible.

Theoretical frameworks

By combining the narrative format with reflexivity, a balance should be found in maintaining the integrity of the nurses' stories and minimising any bias I may have towards the nurses without losing the value of my relationship with them. Most importantly, the analytical tools of narrative, reflexivity and transference create a space within the text where emotion can emerge and be experienced from within the context of the nursing story. Thus, emotion remains central to the whole process. In effect, the analytical tools are used to create a descriptive space in which emotion is shown and in which its embodiment, conscious and unconscious nature and social relevance coexist. Thus, within the narrative, the boundaries of the context are set and in conjunction with the I-It reflexivity, the nursing background is described and emotions that relate to social, cultural and historical phenomena are identified. In conjunction with narrative and I-Thou reflexivity, the individual and social development of relational and communicative emotions also emerge, focusing on individuals' reasoned relationships and their physical embodiment of them. Including transference also provides a representation of the psychodynamic unconscious emergence of emotion. Thus, emotions and emotional experience emerge in the text, which mimics the space between an individual and their environment, while representing their social circumstances, their relationships and their understandings of themselves.

From this point, the nature of the relationship between emotion and emotional labour is explored. Archer's notion of first order emotion is used to help identify the significance for emotional labour of where the emotions are elicited from. Hochschild's notion of feeling rules is used to identify the social manifestation of emotion. Representations of Archer's inner dialogue are also identified and used to examine how emotional labour is linked to self-identity. Bringing these theoretical approaches together, Hochschild's notion of emotion management, feeling rules, surface and deep acting, in respect to emotional labour in nursing, are developed.

Vignette 7 'The complaint'

Emily: Another night shift, I have come home from work this morning feeling really, really, dissatisfied. I got into work and one of the other staff nurses requested that she have a quick word. And in the talk it turns out that one of the patients from the previous night has mentioned to her that she wants to put in a complaint about me. It just made me feel really, really sick. I have never had a complaint made against me. I try not to be rude to the patients. But what happened was that she wanted to go out to the toilet, she's a lady who's quite strong and able to walk and she has had an appendectomy. And I felt that she should walk out to the toilet, and people had been moaning about her that she just languishes in bed and that she hadn't walked out to the toilet during the day. So when she asked for a commode, I said: 'Well, why don't we walk out' she said she didn't feel confident enough to walk out to the toilet, so I said I'll walk with her and explained to her you know, the risk of clots and chest infections, etc. from sitting around in bed. And I didn't feel that I was rude to her at all. We walked out to the toilet and I gave her the buzzer and told her to buzz when she wanted to come back, and I walked back with her from the toilet again. Turns out she felt that I was really rude to her forcing her to walk out, but she told her daughter that I didn't walk with her. Now I found this really frustrating because I made a point of walking with her and walking back and I really, really didn't feel that I was rude to her. So anyway, I felt sick and I felt really upset by it all and I thought I've got to pull myself together. So I went out there and I spoke to the patient regarding the complaint that she wanted to make. It turns out that she was just feeling really fed up. She looks after foster children who were disabled and she was really worried about going home. She felt that she was getting no support from her family. She ended up having a lot of tears and getting very upset and we talked through all her worries, and at the end of it she said that she wasn't going to complain any more, she was really sorry and it wasn't that I was rude, it was just that it was someone making her do something she didn't want to do and she felt that she was being ganged up on by myself and the rest of her family, which is all obviously a little bit weird, you know, but feeling blue post-op she's been through a lot. So in the end something that was a really negative experience at the beginning turned out to be a really positive one. Because I felt that I spent a lot of time with that lady, really talked through her worries and fears and helped to try and solve some of her problems and sort things out for her. But still, I would have rather not gone through it in the first place and I would like to keep my no complaints against me record.

7   Therapeutic emotional labour

Nursing is a significant, therapeutic, interpersonal process. It functions co-operatively with other human processes that make health possible for individuals in communities. In specific situations in which a professional health team offers health services, nurses participate in the organisation of conditions that facilitate natural ongoing tendencies in human organisms. Nursing is an educative instrument, a maturing force that aims to promote forward movement of personality in the direction of creative, constructive, productive, personal, and community living.

(Peplau 1988 [1952]: 16)

Emotional labour is an essential component of nursing care. In this respect, it differs from the emotional labour carried out by flight attendants. In Chapters 7, 8 and 9 emotional labour is shown to be fully integrated within nursing care in three of its primary functions. First, nursing is a therapeutic interpersonal process that aims to promote the health and wellbeing of patients towards independence and the ability to live their lives as fully as possible. Second, nursing involves specialised knowledge, procedures and skills that aim to promote the health and wellbeing of the patient's physical body. Third, nurses work as part of a collaborative interprofessional health care team who bring their combined specialist knowledge together aiming to facilitate their patients along the pathway towards health and wellbeing. Underpinning these functions is an approach towards health that is holistic and educative aiming to assist patients to grow and develop as individuals, as members of their family, community and work or towards the acceptance of death. Different branches of nursing emphasise different aspects of these functions and apply different specialised bodies of knowledge. Fundamental within all these functions however, are good interpersonal communication skills, of which emotional labour is an essential part.

Because individuals are whole people who are not divided into a physical body, a psychological character and a socially interactive person, these different functions of nursing are integrated, and in practice aspects of each may be involved in nursing one patient. For example, Alice Portman, a district nursing sister, gives an excellent example of holistic care when she tells the story of a patient she nursed in the community following prostate surgery.

> I remember one chap I went to, he thought it was the worst thing in the world when he had a catheter in. He locked himself in the house, hid behind the door sort of thing, he couldn't go out, no couldn't possibly go out. He had had his TURP [Trans urethral resectioning of the prostate], um, but he still had a dribbling incontinence. And he wouldn't go out, you know, but his one pleasure was going to the pub and having a drink. So, I had a conversion student with me [enrolled nurse (EN) to RGN] at the time, so I said, 'Come on, we're going to teach this man how to do intermittent self catheterisation, because the important thing in his life is that he can go out and meet his mates, and go to the pub, you know, in the afternoon, at lunch time. This is important to him'. So we taught him. No, he didn't think he could do it, but yes he did! And at the end of the day, he could go out. And in fact we helped him to train himself to become drier and drier and so the need to do the catheterisation became less and less. But it was getting him to believe in himself. And that this wasn't the end of the world, you know, because his world had come to an end because he was stuck with this horrible pipe and he couldn't go out and socialise anymore. So his quality of life, which was important to him, he was able to continue. Just a little episode you know, something that we accept as routine, is far from routine to a person. And can you imagine how you would feel if you had a catheter in? I'd hate it wouldn't you? I can't imagine anything worse.
>
> (Theodosius 1998)

Here the patient had psychological difficulties in adapting to a physiological change in his body. This resulted in him being unable to partake in his normal social activities. In order to promote this patient's health and wellbeing the nurse helped him come to terms with his physiological condition, offering clinical interventions which she taught to the patient alongside continence issues, enabling him to regain his independence. The patient psychologically took control of his condition and worked with the nurse in the management of his continence. He was then able to return to his normal social activities. The nursing care carried out here not only is holistic but also involves a partnership between the nurse and patient. The nurse brought a range of knowledge and skills to that partnership. She used her interpersonal and communication skills to find out about him; she used empathy to help understand his situation; she used her knowledge about continence and her skills in the clinical procedure of catheterisation; she used her ability to teach. Each component of nursing care used here has its own specialist knowledge base, learnt and understood independently even though in the care of this one gentleman they are brought together. In order to understand the nature of emotional labour in nursing, emotional labour has been separated into three aspects: therapeutic, instrumental and collegial. As in the care of this patient, all three aspects of emotional labour may be brought together. These three aspects each have a distinct character linked to three different functions of nursing described earlier. In this chapter emotional labour as an integral part of the therapeutic interpersonal function of nursing is examined. This aspect of emotional labour is called therapeutic emotional labour.

Therapeutic emotional labour

Hildegau Peplau (1988 [1952]) saw the relationship between nurse and patient as being a 'therapeutic' one. She emphasised the interpersonal nature of nursing, focusing on its teaching and counselling roles as vital in promoting patient independence, and facilitating healthy psychological growth and development. Nowadays, patient counselling is usually undertaken by psychotherapists and trained counsellors. Nurses refer or advise patients to access such services rather than counselling themselves. However, the role of listening to patients' concerns and problems, and providing a safe place in which they can express their feelings and adjust to changes taking place in their lives, is still an important part of nursing care. As noted in Chapter 2, being able to express one's feelings in such situations is believed to have therapeutic value. That the patient can do so in the presence of the nurse is an important feeling rule.

The role of education in nursing is readily recognised as today it is fundamental to health promotion. However, it has been a part of the nurse's role since Florence Nightingale (1980 [1859]) first advocated it. The belief behind

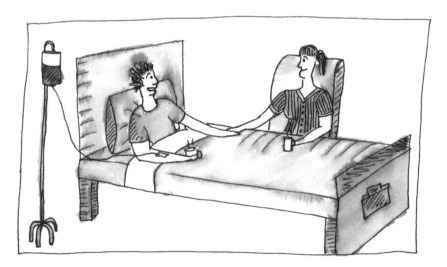

'Exchanging confidences'

patient education is that being equipped with relevant information enables them to take greater responsibility in promoting and maintaining their own health. Thus, the hope is that individuals will see the importance of the information to their health and act to promote it; it is a health care value.

Education and counselling often go together. In order to enable the patient to psychologically adapt to their changed circumstances (temporary or otherwise), information about what is happening to them and the reasons behind their care are given. The patient's role in this process is not a passive one; it is participatory. Unless the patient chooses to participate, the care cannot be forced on to them without them being sectioned under the Mental Health Care Act. A central purpose of the nurse's role is to facilitate the patient to adapt, to cooperate with, and ultimately to take responsibility for that care. Thus patient independence is encouraged in a way that facilitates their psychological growth and development so that they themselves can act to promote their own health and wellbeing. The personality and the ability of the patient to participate in this relationship therefore is a contributory factor. Thus, Peplau notes:

> in every contact with another human being there is the *possibility* for the nurse of working toward common understandings and goals; every contact between two human beings involves the *possibility* of a clash of feelings, beliefs and ways of acting.
>
> (Peplau 1988: xi, my emphasis)

Peplau maintains that the kind of person the nurse is contributes towards how the patient relates to them, and consequently receives the care offered. Thus, Peplau believed that in order for the nurse to be able to enter into an interpersonal therapeutic relationship, she needs to be self-aware because she has a professional obligation to bring her knowledge and skill to that relationship:

> Being able to understand one's own behaviour, to help others to identify difficulties and to apply principles of human relations to the problems that arise at all levels of experience – these are functions of nursing.
>
> (Peplau 1988: xi)

In order to establish and build an interpersonal and therapeutic relationship between herself and the patient, the nurse needs to be able to manage her own emotions for the benefit of the patient. In order to do so, she needs to be aware of her own feelings, the patient's feelings, and have an awareness of how these might impact on the patient in the moment of their interaction, and in meeting the nursing goals. This kind of emotion management is what I term *therapeutic emotional labour* (see Table 7.1).

Therapeutic emotional labour (TEL) is therefore where the nursing intention is to enable the establishment or maintenance of the interpersonal

Table 7.1 Therapeutic emotional labour

Purpose	Emotions	Skills	Feeling rules
The establishment and/or maintenance of the therapeutic relationship between nurse and patient.	Subject–subject emotions related to self-worth.	Interpersonal communication skills.	Education facilitates patient understanding of health care needs.
		Self-reflexivity.	The nurse cares for the patient's psychological wellbeing.
To facilitate patient cooperation with care offered.			Confiding and expressing anxieties to the nurse is therapeutic.
To encourage the patient to take responsibility for their own health and wellbeing.			The nurse can facilitate a peaceful and dignified death.

therapeutic relationship between nurse and patient in order to promote the psychological and emotional wellbeing of the patient in a way that facilitates their movement towards independent healthy living. TEL is dealing with emotions that are directly concerned with expressions of self-worth and personal identity of both the patient and the nurse, elicited from their interactive relationship (subject–subject relations: see Table 5.1, page 93). TEL may involve giving patients appropriate information on which they can act. This is predicated on the belief that health education is essential to individuals taking responsibility for their own health care needs. TEL may involve the nurse encouraging the patient to express and talk about their feelings and concerns while managing their own emotions. It is predicated on the belief that disclosure and discussion of personal and private problems is therapeutic for the patient, and within nursing, is typical of emotional labour represented in the Nightingale Ethic. TEL may involve both the nurse and patient accepting the inevitability of death, predicated on the belief that the nurse can facilitate the patient towards as peaceful and dignified a death as possible.

Therapeutic emotional labour in 'The complaint' (Vignette 7)

Vignette 7 is taken from the audio diary of Emily, an E grade staff nurse in the alpha popular subgroup. Emily was an exceptionally good nurse: her knowledge and clinical and communication skills were well recognised by everyone on the ward. Although the story in this vignette is about a patient's complaint, unfortunately a common occurrence in nursing nowadays, the emotional labour carried out here is therapeutic. In TEL, the nurse works towards establishing an interpersonal relationship; in this case this involved the nurse working beyond a clash of feelings and beliefs between her and her patient. Through her emotional labour, Emily created a space in which more meaningful communication could take place. The patient was able to express her feelings and concerns, and therapeutic value was gained from this as she felt better for doing so. This is not a romanticised example of the nurse coming along and making the patient feel better through her natural caring abilities however. Both parties had to work on their emotions.

The boundaries

This story is clearly about two people, Emily and the patient. It is a story about their feelings in respect to a nursing interaction which brought them together. The motivation and impetus to this particular encounter are negative emotions. In relation to Archer's (2000) emotion orders, the first order emotions elicited and the second order emotions that emerge from the encounter are concerned with self-worth and personal identity.

Emily's emotions motivate her to defend herself against the patient's complaint about her. She sees the complaint as impinging on her sense of identity and self-worth because it shames her in the eyes of others. Emily mentions twice that she has not previously had a complaint made against her; in fact, only two nurses on the ward had a no-complaints record. Her no-complaints record was a source of pride. She was proud of her ability to communicate and listen fairly to all people. She considered herself easy to get on with and was overtly friendly. Emily was known and respected on the ward for her ease of manner and camaraderie with people. This understanding of herself mattered to her. For example, in an earlier entry in her diary, Emily comments that the other staff nurse on nights with her, had told her:

> I really enjoy working with you, you don't take over, you let me get on with it but you are there for support. That made me feel really good because that's exactly the way I like to come across to people and that I support them and that I don't take over and also coming from her that's really good because she always says what she thinks and I like that.

Emily therefore sees the complaint as a personal attack against her personal integrity and her sense of identity. The attack made her feel sick. Her reaction is similar to the flight/fight response to a threatening stimulus. However, Emily chooses to fight back rather than withdraw because she believes that the complaint is unjustified, suggesting that she was also experiencing anger, secondary to the shame (Lewis 1971; Scheff 1990). Her feelings are reflexively managed in two ways. First, it is her emotional distress that motivates her to confront the patient; second, although these feelings are motivational, she suppresses them in her interaction with the patient. Emily is obviously very good at surface acting because the patient does not appear to feel threatened by her challenge. However, the patient is not deceived about Emily's feelings either because she knows that the basis on which she is making the complaint is unjustified.

The patient's anger is provoked by her perception that Emily failed to respond to her anxiety and made her walk out to the toilet. This anger initiates the complaint and subsequent interaction with Emily. Her complaint is also arguably a cry for help in the belief that the nurse might recognise this and be concerned for her patient. The patient is anxious that due to her ill health she may not be able to fulfil her responsibilities as a mother on her return home, threatening her self-worth as a good mother. These emotions motivate her to put in a complaint about Emily. Lupton (1996) notes that patient perceptions of what constitutes a good or bad doctor, are created by the doctor's ability to pick up on personal, emotional distress that may lie behind the patient's physical symptoms. It is possible that the patient is angry at Emily for not realising that her reluctance to walk out to the bathroom was due to other emotional factors causing her distress. In her eyes Emily is a bad nurse.

Dynamic tensions

There is an existing tension between Emily and the patient as a result of the initial interaction. Underlying this is a tension between two different feeling rules, both integral to TEL. First, the relationship was originally established when Emily assists her patient in walking out to the bathroom. Emily explains that following surgery, patients are at risk from developing clots and chest infections: this is why the nurses are suggesting that she walks out to the toilet. Emily establishes why it is important patients walk out to the bathroom and by walking there and back with her, acknowledges her anxiety by giving her reassurance and support. Emily acts within her role mediated by feeling rules identified earlier in which she educates the patient about the care given. She also asserts control over the patient's body in a way that both reflects her knowledge and expertise in looking after post-operative patients and demonstrates care and concern for the patient. In this action a degree of trust and an attachment has been established between them.

The patient in her role expresses her reluctance, but cooperates and walks out to the bathroom. There is no 'rational' reason why she should not cooperate. However, the patient feels as if she has no control, for by explaining why she must walk out to the toilet, Emily has taken away her reason not to. In addition, Emily has not provided a space in which her patient can confess her worries: she has not discerned the *real* reason for her reluctance. The patient consequently feels as if she is being 'ganged up on'. The patient needs to find a way in which she can reassert control and make Emily listen to her. Ideology behind patient's right to complain is concerned with allowing individuals to express their feelings and opinions, in order to influence the health care provided. It enables a degree of self-expression. The difficulty with this, as Craib (1994) points out, is that in order to have this kind of influence, the individual needs to know what it is they want to say and what they want to happen as a result of it. 'Of course' Craib (1994: 121) comments, 'if we are really going to be in charge of our own lives, then we are going to need to manipulate others into giving us what we want from them'. The patient's initiation of a complaint is a clear attempt to manipulate Emily; however, the basis for it is inaccurate as she is actually struggling to express her feelings. Thus the reason she gives is that she felt that her own control had been taken away from her. In order to express this, she lodges an unfair complaint against Emily, a nurse to whom she has an attachment and, therefore, is in a position to manipulate. This is a gamble. Some nurses would have walked away from the situation and not attempted to resolve it as Emily did.

Growth

Following the complaint, their interaction becomes more personal reflecting their personal identity (as individuals) rather than their social identity (as a generic nurse and patient). By making the complaint Emily's patient forces her to deal with her as a particular individual who is grappling with the fact that her illness has brought added complications to her life, rather than changed her previous responsibilities. By confronting the patient about her complaint, Emily forces the patient to deal with her personally, for Emily knows that she was not rude to the patient. Their relationship is not entirely happy. Emily is confused and hurt by the patient's accusations: although she carries out TEL by suppressing her own feelings and listens to the patient's fears, she quite clearly does not fully understand why they should cause her to put in a complaint. Consequently, Emily falls back on the patient's sick role by noting her vulnerability due to her operation; in doing so she re-establishes the patient's role in relation to her own as the nurse. The patient withdraws the complaint, not because her problems are now solved, but because someone has listened: Emily is now acting according to her expected role.

Emily's TEL and the patient's emotion expressions are directly concerned with their individual perceptions of their personal identity; both of them fear that their self-worth is being eroded. In the communication that subsequently takes place, the patient reveals that her concern is that she will be unable to successfully undertake her duties as a foster mother and that this will bring disapprobation. Her reluctance to walk out to the bathroom, in her insistence that she is unable to, is an action that is meant to say, 'I am sick, therefore, I have a legitimate reason for being unable to fulfil my duties'. The introduction of the role her relatives play is important to this discourse for she mentions that they too were 'ganging up' on her.

In making the complaint, the action of the patient makes Emily vulnerable to her. This suggests that there is a degree of transference occurring because in doing so, she brings disapprobation to Emily. Mutual trust becomes an integral part of the communication process. By confronting the patient, Emily exposes herself to further potential denigration of her character. By admitting her wrongdoing and expressing her real concerns, the patient also makes herself vulnerable to Emily. Although the trust between the two has been challenged, it does exist because the patient tells Emily her real fears and Emily listens and accepts even if she does not understand. In fact, Emily sees their discussion as representing a positive TEL experience because she believes in the feeling rule that talking about worries and anxieties is helpful.

Possibilities

This vignette highlights the relationship between social conditioning and normative expectations of culturally defined roles, such as that of nurse and patient, juxtaposed with expressions of emotion concerned with the emergence of personal identity. It demonstrates the interactive, relational nature of emotional labour and it shows how, in this case, the emotions managed through TEL are concerned with self-worth. What does this reveal about the nature of TEL in nursing today?

Towards the end of Vignette 7, Emily makes an enlightening comment:

> So in the end something that was a really negative experience at the beginning turned out to be a really positive one. Because I felt that I spent a lot of time with that lady, really talked through her worries and fears and helped to try and solve some of her problems and sort things out for her. But still, I would have rather not gone through it in the first place and I would like to keep my no complaints against me record.

Emily acknowledges that the encounter represents a good nurse–patient therapeutic interaction, in that through her TEL and good communication skills, the patient talked through her feelings and felt better; but still, she would have preferred not to have had to do this. For Emily, the incident is representative of her; it is not just a generic nurse–patient interaction. It is through this relationship that the role and emergence of personal identity can be seen in emotional labour.

Emily's inner dialogue is revealing here. Her internal conversation is based around the 'I' of the present and her 'me' representing her overall self drawn from past experiences. However, the 'you' an appeal to the future self appears to be missing from the dialogue. This suggests that Emily is choosing not to give this incidence importance from which she can grow and assess her future self and possible responses. She reaches the dedication phase where the overall cost is assessed without the need to project into the future; the cost to her self is possibly too high.

Autonomy and the investment of self in therapeutic emotional labour

Archer writes:

> In addition to there being a normative order, we the subjects have to care about it, or at least about some of it. For social evaluations to matter – and without mattering they are incapable of generating emotionality – they have to gel with our concerns . . . Such concerns . . . are socially forged out of subjects' reflections upon what is important to them in their ineluctably social lives . . . 'Our feelings of shame, remorse, pride, dignity, moral obligations, aspirations to excel, just because the imports they involve are essentially those of a subject, all incorporate a sense of what is important to us in our lives as subjects' [Taylor 1985: 54].
>
> (Archer 2000: 219)

Being the object of a complaint is a matter of concern for Emily. It impacts on her sense of personal identity, and therefore on her feelings concerned with her self-worth. This has been said before; but it is crucial to understanding the nature of Emily's emotional labour. She has carried out her nursing duty well, succeeding in walking the patient out to the toilet where other nurses failed. Yet now, a formal complaint is being submitted about her and she is infused with shame, frustration and anxiety as her character is brought into disrepute. The intensity of this makes her feel sick to her stomach. Denzin comments that:

> Emotion is a lived, believed in, situated, temporally embodied experience that radiates through a person's stream of consciousness, is felt in, and runs through, his [sic] body, and in the process of being lived, plunges the person and his associates into a wholly new and transformed reality of a world that is being constituted by the emotional experience.
>
> (Denzin 1984: 66)

Emily's reality has been transformed; the experience entirely dominates her perception of the night shift. When she returns home and describes the shift in her audio diary she begins by stating how dissatisfied she *is still* feeling, after having dealt with the situation and admitting that the interaction was ultimately a positive one. She is still distressed and upset by the incident. In fact, unlike her previous entries in the diary, she mentions no other events in the shift at all. It matters immensely because she takes pride in having a no-complaints record, in having good communication skills and in how she carries out her duties as a nurse. In fact, she is meticulous about it. This is why she asserts so strenuously that she made a point of walking out to the toilet and back again with her patient. It is because it matters that she chooses to defend herself and confront the patient. Katz (1999) notes that it is through the social framework and normative structures that personal characteristics can be acted out, and when those are made evident to an individual or called into question it can elicit 'spiritual' shame as their actions, normally embedded, natural and inherent become obvious, overt and under scrutiny:

> Personal identity everywhere is an achieved performance of ascriptive characteristics. One learns how to enact fundamental features of personal identity in ways that suggest that the features are inherent, natural, matters of grace and not products of years of culturally guided practice . . . Any line of social action, from casual conversation to an artistic performance to a sexual interaction, is vulnerable to breakdown from too-close attention to its necessary machinations. Awkwardness, not just practical ignorance, threatens to provoke destructive shame. But the alternative is not the transcendence of shame. A constant running on the surface of shame is a necessary foundation of social action.
>
> (Katz 1999: 170–171)

In other words, Emily's aspiration to excel as a nurse is called into question, eliciting shame and damaging her pride. Her personal identity is vulnerable to breakdown from too close attention to it. In order to restore her dignity she needs to be seen to be vindicated. Thus, on the surface, shame propels Emily into defending her previous actions in the initial encounter when she walked the patient to the toilet. On a deeper lever, her action protects her sense of personal identity. This vindicates actions that she considers natural and inherent in her projection of self through her social identity as a nurse who is a good communicator, friendly and caring of her patient's needs – essential components of her personal identity.

TEL, carried out as an interactive process, draws on a 'sense of self that is considered integral' (Hochschild 1983: 15) and has many layers. One layer of the interaction is visible when each woman becomes vulnerable to the other, and a degree of trust is established based on feeling rules as a result of their interaction. The emotional labour becomes a therapeutic encounter: an encounter shaped by social norms concerned with the Nightingale Ethic but challenged by changing attitudes towards consumer rights, customer care and patient satisfaction. A further layer of the interaction is that each individual is acting to protect their sense of self-worth and personal integrity, both forging a space in which the patient's emotions can emerge, and a therapeutic outcome is achieved. For Emily, however, there is another layer of interaction, in that she holds back from reidentifying herself with her nursing role and projection of self as a good communicator, even though she quite clearly demonstrates this. Her comment that she would rather not have gone through the process at all indicates her need to separate herself from the incident. Her attitude is similar to Buber's 'I-It' attitude (Jacoby 1984), even though she initiates the second encounter, and through her emotional labour evokes a therapeutic outcome, and vindicating herself in the process. Emily *needs* to separate herself from the encounter in order to feel vindicated. To move into the 'I-Thou' relationship she would have to relate to the genuine otherness of her patient, which she evidently does not. She retains her personal identity as distinct from the generic nursing one, while enabling the patient, through her emotional labour, to forge a therapeutic relationship with the idea of the good nurse, creating a comfortable space in which she can confess her real concerns and feelings.

The nature of therapeutic emotional labour in nursing

Emotional labour in nursing is needed by patients because they are vulnerable; which implicates it in mediating power and trust between the nurse and the patient. Louise de Raeve (2002) infers that nurses consequently have a moral responsibility towards their patients.

> Nurses are not serving customers as flight attendants do, they are responding to the needs of vulnerable, often frightened and suffering people who are partially, or totally dependent on their help. These facts, combined with the power imbalance between nurses and patients, and the trust that patients generally have in nurses behove nurses to try not to act harshly towards patients, but to subject to self reflective enquiry any negative, premature judgements that initial emotional reactions may precipitate. In this respect, at least I would want to claim that a nurse's impetus towards a deepening of his or her understanding and compassion could have nothing to do with acting, whether 'deep' or otherwise. The consequences of thinking that it does are utterly counterintuitive.
>
> (de Raeve 2002: 470)

It is essential that nurses carry out self-reflective enquiry in respect to TEL. This is because not only do nurses have a moral responsibility towards their patients, but also it is vital to their own personal growth and therefore, to their ability to carry out effective TEL in meeting this responsibility. However, because TEL is an interactive and relational encounter between nurse and patient, the personal identities of both the *patient* and the nurse are involved. Thus, patients are also implicated in this moral responsibility. The nurse's responsibility and growth therefore need to be considered in this context.

For example, in Vignette 7, Emily does not demonstrate self-reflection that enables her to extend compassion towards the patient. She does not extend compassion because she does not empathise with the patient. Rather she excuses the patient's behaviour on the basis that she is unwell. She comments that it 'is all obviously a little bit weird, you know, but feeling blue post-op she's been through a lot'. This is not because Emily is uncaring or unkind. Nor is it because her TEL is inauthentic. Rather it is because Emily chooses not to follow through her self-reflection and project into the future and learn from this experience. For example, she does not ask herself why she did not use the opportunity to ask her what was really troubling her when walking the patient to and from the toilet. This lack of self-reflection is surprising because Emily prides herself on her good communication skills, which she obviously has as she successfully brings this situation to a therapeutic resolution for the patient.

Peplau (1988 [1952]) argues that the personality of the nurse affects the relationship she forms with the patient, which consequently affects their experience of their care. However, she goes on to say:

> Concepts, principles, skills and abilities can be said to be learned when new behaviour follows examination and discussion of problems that require particular principles and skills in their resolution. Thus . . . *fostering personality development in the direction of maturity is a function of nursing and nursing education; it requires the use of principles and methods that permit and guide the process of grappling with everyday interpersonal problems or difficulties.*
>
> (Peplau 1988: x, original emphasis)

As Hochschild (1983) establishes, teaching and monitoring emotional labour is an important part of it. Smith (1992) particularly emphasised this point: nurses need to be taught emotional labour. Understanding the nature of emotional labour and how it relates to the self is absolutely essential to this process. It is not enough to say that the nurse needs to suppress what she really feels and express a more appropriate emotion in its place. Nor is it sufficient to say that she should imagine what the patient might be feeling in order to facilitate deep acting. Emotions are not that easily managed and because they reflect aspects of the self that are considered integral, they have consequences. For example, Susan in Vignette 4 'The murderer' had done her utmost to care for her patient in a highly stressful situation. In a shared decision with other health care professionals, it was decided that the patient would not be resuscitated in the future. The patient's sister responded to this by accusing Susan of murdering her sister. 'I felt like a murderer. I felt guilty and it was horrible.' How was Susan supposed to manage such emotions? The student nurse advised her, 'Don't worry about it, forget it.' Susan's succinct response to the suggestion that she should suppress or repress her emotions is: 'You haven't got a clue . . . I am responsible for her.' Susan accepted that she has a moral responsibility towards her patient and her patient's sister. Similarly, Emily accepts that she has a moral responsibility towards her patient. In order to extend empathy towards the patient's sister Susan also tried using her imagination even to the extent that she was begging the patient not to die: 'I was going, "*Please* hold on for your sister" . . . I really was begging her to hold on because I knew that once her sister got there and saw what a state she was in, she would agree to the NFR status.' However, her empathy and her use of her imagination did not help *Susan* deal with the emotional trauma.

Dealing with emotional difficulties is common in nursing. They are not always concerned with emergency situations like Susan's; they can be concerned with routine nursing, like Emily's situation in Vignette 7, or they can develop over a long period of time as with Alix's family in Vignette 2. As de Raeve (2002) points out nurses are not serving customers; they are responding to the needs of people who are under their care because they are vulnerable. Thus, it is the moral responsibility of the nursing profession to find a way to equip its nurses to manage their emotions in a way that as Peplau (1988: x) asserts fosters the development of personality in the direction of maturity. To do this, nurses need to understand the process of emotion management as it relates to self-reflection more fully. In Chapters 9 and 10 the process of emotion management is explored in more detail.

The process of emotional labour, however, involves two people. The behaviour, attitudes and actions of the patients and relatives contribute towards that relationship. In Vignette 2, Alix's dad was verbally aggressive and physically intimidating; in Vignette 4, the sister was verbally abusive towards Susan; and in Vignette 7, the patient manipulates Emily by making a complaint about her. Of course, these people are vulnerable and in pain. But does this mean that the nurses who care for them can be treated like punch bags just because it is their job to carry out 'emotional labour' as if it is a commodity? Nurses are people who also have feelings and a right to expect their human dignity to be respected. TEL requires the nurse to bring something that is integral to herself to the relationship with the patient. In Emily's example her sense of self was brought into disrepute. Consequently she worked to protect herself by vindicating her actions. In this situation, the patient should not have needed to manipulate the nurse into providing a space where she can confess her feelings of anxiety. The responsibility for this is Emily's. Equally, however, Emily should not have had to experience a denigration of her character just so that the patient can tell her how she is feeling. The responsibility for this is the patient's. The moral responsibility therefore is *shared*. Nurses are serving the community, but they are also members of it. They try to meet the needs of vulnerable people, but in doing so make themselves vulnerable to them.

In meeting the nursing responsibility, the profession perhaps needs to consider why Emily failed to ask her patient why she was reluctant to walk out to the toilet. One of the difficulties with TEL is that it is often seen as being separate from nursing care, partly because nursing care is considered as clinical, and partly because the psychological needs of patients are now the responsibility of counsellors and psychiatrists. Why Emily failed to identify her patient's real feelings and the changing nature of nursing care is considered in Chapter 8. Instrumental emotional labour, an aspect of emotional labour that is integral to the clinical role of nursing, is introduced and explored.

Vignette 8 'The NG tube'

Catherine: What about the skill side of it, the clinical side, do you enjoy that, or is it just the communication side?

Kate: The clinical side, I think, is something that should come after you have learnt how to behave with people. I think that [the clinical side] is something that you can learn once you know how to be a nurse. And now I feel that I'm just learning that and I've done nursing since I was 18 [was HCA previously]. I might only have been qualified for a year but I feel that there is so much more to learn that I feel quite receptive to what I'm learning, that I will always ask. I always want to know how I'm doing things and if I'm doing it right and once I know how I'm doing something, I still check up and make sure that I'm doing it right. Even if I know it inside out I'll go to somebody and say, 'Look, I'm taking a CVP [central venous pressure] line out, I do it like this don't I?' and they go, 'Yeah, yeah all right, off you go!' But in my mind I like to know that I'm doing it right. And then if I'm doing it right, then I can go and do it in a relaxed manner with the patient, put them at ease, and they don't even know half the time that things are being done.

Do you think that's the real skill?

Yeah, it's the art of science. One example is before I was qualified I'd never put an NG [naso-gastric] tube down, and I've only put two down since I qualified in August. The first one I did – I had seen loads of them being put down, I had done the theory behind it – I knew what I had to do but I had never actually done it on my own at all, or with help or anything. So I had somebody that needed an NG tube down, so I didn't have any choice, I had to do it. I asked one of the senior staff nurses to talk me through it now, and then to come and check on me in about five or ten minutes and see how I was getting on. This NG tube went in like a dream. This patient didn't even know that I'd never done it before. And he relaxed because I said, 'I'm going to do this and I'm going to do that, you're going to have a swallow for me, here is some nice cold water' and all the rigmarole that you go through and afterwards he said, 'Cor that was easy!' I said, 'I know!' [*laughs in astonishment*] 'It was easy for me too!' And he said, 'Why, you must have done hundreds of these!' and I said, 'No that was my first one!' And he went, 'Blimey I didn't know'. And then the second NG tube I put down somebody, I had a student with me. So I went to a senior nurse and checked that I was doing it the right way in my head and then I went and talked it through with my student – all the time

I believe in reinforcing what I'm doing – so I talked it through with my student, then went and did it with the patient, put the NG down. Got it sorted out. He actually pulled it out, he didn't like it, and he pulled it out within about five minutes of it being down. So I said, 'Fair enough, that's it. I'm not going to do it again, it's obviously distressed you', so I told the doctors. I had a bit of reflection time with my student at the end of the shift. And I said to her, 'How many NG tubes do you think I've put down?' Because I was trying to get across to her the fact you've got to relax patients and be at ease even if you don't really know what you're doing, because she was a very nervous girl and she said, 'Um I don't know, you've probably done hundreds'. And I said, 'That was my second one, and I was as nervous as you were and as he was you know', and she said, 'I'd have never have known'. So even though I had butterflies in my stomach, on the outside I was trying to put across that I did know what I was doing.

So you were like sort of controlling your own emotions for the benefit of yourself, the benefit of the patient and for the benefit of the student?

Yes. I think so, because you can't do your job if you're fingers and thumbs and you don't know what you're doing. So you have to have a certain amount of control over what you're doing yourself, and I think that is a part of the art of it, really, the art of doing what we do.

When you did that NG tube with that student, how did it make you feel when you achieved what you set out to achieve?

I don't know, because I got it down, and he pulled it out and I had to get on with the next thing! No, I had done what I had to do for him and he pulled it out. I told the doctors that this man can't have an NG tube, if you want it, put it down yourself, and then I went on to the next job because I was working with fifteen patients, with only one student, me and one HCA.

So you didn't really reflect on the success of it and feel satisfaction for it?

Not at the time, no. Oh, I don't know, I mean I've used it as an example, but I didn't really feel, 'Oh brilliant I've done that'. I just think well it's another thing I've got under my belt, move on to the next thing. You know, I pocket things, you know, file them away. I've learnt one thing, I've learnt it, I've done it once, done it twice, done it three times, right I feel confident competent at it. I just log it away, and then the next time I do something new, do it once, twice and again and feel confident and I log it away. And it all gets filed and I suppose you just increase your skill mix don't you as you are learning more and more things and that should be happening all the time and you should be learning something every day.

Do you think you feel satisfaction in increasing the amount you know rather than thinking about the satisfaction of specific things?

Yes, exactly, that is how I feel. I'd rather have the increase in knowledge than have the satisfaction of doing individual things, I feel more satisfied at the end of a shift knowing that I have done as much as possible in the time that I have got and the patients that I have got. I have stopped coming home feeling dissatisfied, less so I should say, because of the fact I wasn't able to get my job done before, but now, because I know for a fact that I never sit down, I don't ever stop. I am always on the move doing one thing or another and even if that is just sitting on a bed just talking to a patient who is frightened about going for an op or is emotional about something, that to me all needs doing. If a dressing doesn't get done because I have been talking to a patient or a relative, then it does not get done. Because it is 24 hour care and I am learning to adapt to that because it is what needs doing now, it's what I put my priorities in.

8 Instrumental emotional labour

In general nursing, clinical nursing skills and competencies linked to the biomedical model are essential to nursing practice. This is particularly the case in surgical nursing where patients come into hospital to have invasive physiological procedures. Surgery is a direct action that sets out to correct problems in the body by cutting, bypassing, removing or replacing. These actions interfere with normal bodily functions and nursing care is aimed at preparing the patient prior to theatre and facilitating the body's healing and reparation processes afterwards. The nurse's knowledge of anatomy and physiology of the healthy body, the impact of surgery on the body, and the clinical skills involved in supporting the body's normal functions and dealing with complications arising as a result of surgery are fundamental to the care given. This is the case for all surgical procedures. However, not all patients are fit and healthy prior to theatre. They may come in with existing known or unknown conditions. The nurse also needs to be knowledgeable about the impact of different illnesses on the body and how the treatments given work. For example, a patient may come in to have an amputation of a limb due to complications of diabetes. The nurse must also manage the patient's diabetes, which will be affected as a result of the surgery. While the clinical procedures related to surgery (or indeed other forms of nursing) may be routine to the nurse, for the patient they can appear formidable, provoking anxiety at a time when they might already be enduring a great deal of pain and stress. Instrumental emotional labour is an aspect of emotional labour that supports the clinical and medical knowledge base of nursing practice in the execution of clinical skills. This chapter examines the instrumental character of emotional labour in nursing.

Instrumental emotional labour

Instrumental emotional labour (IEL) is carried out as *a direct result of* a clinical nursing intervention. The motivation for the labour therefore is instrumental. It is an example of *Zweckrational*, or goal-orientated action (Weber in Gerth and Mills 1991). Its purpose is to successfully facilitate the clinical nursing procedure in a way that minimises pain and discomfort and maximises the healing process of the patient's physical body. This is a twofold process. First, IEL aims to relax the patient's body in order that a physically invasive clinical procedure can be successfully carried out. It is concerned with managing patient emotions of anxiety and fear elicited from the body–environment relationship in the natural order (see Table 5.1, page 93). The feeling rule concerned with IEL is predicated on the belief that a relaxed, receptive frame of mind can impact on the physical body by relaxing it. Second, IEL is also carried out to produce the proper state of mind in the nurse as well as the patient. This is to facilitate her performative skill in efficiently carrying out the task. Emotions elicited and managed here are from the practical order and concerned with subject–object relations (see Table 5.1). The feeling rule associated with the nurse's emotion state is predicated on the belief that relaxing her own body and eliciting confidence in her skills enables her to perform the task better thereby minimising the patient's discomfort. How the emotions connect to personal identity in the interaction that occurs between the nurse and the patient in IEL is different from that of TEL. In IEL the emotions experienced by the patient are concerned with the potential threat to his physical body. The patient is therefore concerned with his personal safety. The emotions elicited from the nurse are concerned with her performative achievement in her skill and clinical competency, and thus are directly concerned with her evaluation of her skills in respect to her identity as a nurse. Because IEL stems from a social interaction between the nurse and patient, emotions are also elicited from the social order (see Table 5.1). The patient puts his trust in the nurse's ability to efficiently carry out the clinical procedure in a way that both acknowledges his anxieties and minimalises any pain and discomfort he may experience. The nurse uses her interpersonal skills to make this process as comfortable as possible. This makes the patient feel secure and cared for – his sense of self-worth confirmed in feeling valued. In return for her skill and care, the patient offers gratitude to the nurse – who feels pride, her sense of self-worth confirmed in doing something valuable for others (see Table 8.1).

Instrumental emotional labour in 'The NG tube' (Vignette 8)

Vignette 8, 'The NG tube', is taken from Kate, a D grade staff nurse's interview. At the beginning of the participant observation, Kate had just qualified. This was her first staffing post as a qualified nurse. The interview took place a year after she had qualified. In the vignette she describes how she learnt to pass naso-gastric tubes and in doing so illustrates the importance of IEL to the successful accomplishment of clinical procedures.

Boundaries

Kate tells two stories in order to answer the question posed at the beginning of the vignette, and illustrate her point. There are effectively three stories

Table 8.1 Instrumental emotional labour

Purpose	Emotions	Skills	Feeling rules
To minimise patient discomfort and pain due to an invasive procedure. To facilitate patient cooperation with clinical procedures. To facilitate the nurse's clinical competency.	Body–environment emotions related to physiological wellbeing and safety. Subject–object emotions related to performative achievement and personal identity. Subject–subject emotions related to self worth.	Interpersonal communication skills. Performative clinical skills.	A calm receptive mind can relax the physiological body thereby reducing pain and discomfort. A calm and receptive mind enables the nurse to perform clinical skills efficiently and competently. A relaxed nurse promotes confidence in her patient's expectation of her clinical competency. The patient can trust the nurse's clinical skill, and care of their probable anxiety.

inside each other. The outside story is the conversation between Kate and me; this is concerned with the wider nursing debate about the relationship between nurses' interpersonal and clinical skills – the art and science of nursing. The inside stories illustrate this discussion but are stories in their own right, both being good examples of IEL. The inside stories and what they reveal about the nature of IEL are examined first, and then the wider context in which IEL is situated is considered.

Kate explains the importance of good interpersonal skills in carrying out clinical tasks and procedures well, which she sees as being about her confidence and ability in her clinical skills, rather than in her communication skills. She points out the importance of feeling confident in the knowledge and technical procedure involved in the task. This assurance frees the nurse to focus on her patient's worries because she is in control, confident that she can perform the procedure well. The understanding that nurses need to manage their own emotions in order to maximise their ability to perform a skill without too much thought, freeing up their ability to concentrate on the patient's experience, is a view of their role that is readily recognised and accepted. To illustrate this, Kate describes the first two occasions she inserted an NG tube. It is important to note, that Kate draws on her initial learning experiences to demonstrate her point. This is because once ease of competency has been achieved and the nurse routinely feels satisfied with her performance, it becomes pre-reflexive. She does not need to think about how she is managing her own emotions in respect to the task. It does not make this part of the IEL less relevant, however. Emotions elicited from the practical order are important to personal identity in respect to the individual's abilities and consequently, to the social roles they chose to invest themselves in (Archer 2000). Because Kate is newly qualified, she gives an insight into the importance of this.

Dynamic tensions

Kate has a patient who requires an NG tube inserting: she has to carry out this procedure even though she never has done before. She has learnt the theory and observed the procedure as a student, but has no direct practical experience. Kate needs to find a way to carry out this procedure without the patient knowing that she has never done it before, because the patient needs to have confidence in his nurse. This is the crux of the story. First, Kate sets out to prepare herself for the task. She makes sure that in her own mind she knows exactly what she is going to do and why. She also ensures her patient's safety by asking the senior nurse to check on her to make certain everything is going well. Second, as she carries out the task she explains what she is doing to the patient throughout, eliciting his cooperation in the task. She says: 'And he relaxed because I said, "I'm going to do this and I'm going to do that, you're going to have a swallow for me, here is some nice cold water" and all the rigmarole that you go through.' The NG tube goes in easily; both nurse and patient are relieved. Kate experiences satisfaction at a task she has accomplished well, the patient is relieved that it was not quite the awful experience he was expecting. Then, as the patient expresses his gratitude, Kate confesses that she has never done this before and the patient congratulates her, assuring her he had no idea. Thus, Kate's IEL has been a complete success. She has managed her own emotions and the patient's.

Kate describes the second occasion she inserted an NG tube to reinforce the importance of the IEL carried out. She creates extra emphasis because of the role of the student nurse. Her preparation of the task is essential to this:

> you can't do your job if you're fingers and thumbs and you don't know what you are doing. So you have to have a certain amount of control over what you're doing yourself, and I think that is a part of the art of it, really, the art of what we do.

This is a significant point, which returns the stories back to the conversation that is taking place in the interview. Peplau (1988) asserts that how the nurse handles herself is crucial to how she interacts with her patient. Kate suggests

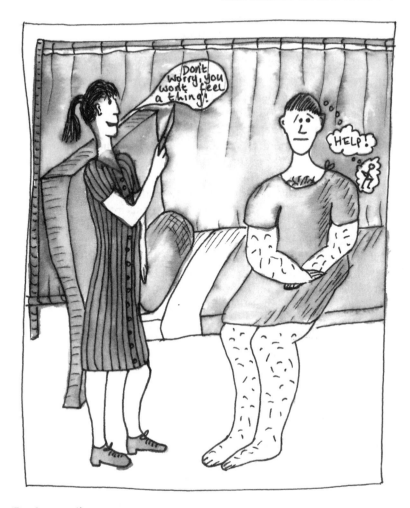

'Don't worry!'

that this is especially the case when performing clinical skills. In fact, she argues that without this knowledge, one cannot effectively do so. This is the point Chapter 7 arrived at, except in this case the focus of the emotional labour is instrumental to the clinical task; whereas Emily's emotional labour was therapeutic, its focus being her patient's psychological wellbeing.

Growth

Growth occurs incrementally as Kate's knowledge and confidence in her abilities and in her role increases. She consolidates each new skill she learns, by practising it until she is confident in it. This is made easier by the fact that the IEL that accompanies each skill is one that as a profession, nursing is well versed in. As each new skill is introduced, IEL is taught as a crucial component of it. Kate demonstrates this in the lesson she gives to her student: 'So even though I had butterflies in my stomach, on the outside I was trying to put across that I did know what I was doing'. Kate's reference to 'that rigmarole' refers to the little tricks and means taught to nurses so that they can help their patients to relax pertinent muscles. NG tubes are passed through the nose down the oesophagus into the stomach; it is a distinctly unpleasant experience. The body reacts by trying to expel it by regurgitation. Anxiety about the procedure results in the muscles in the oesophagus tightening and reinforces the idea that the tube is unwanted. The sensation of an object in your throat is hard to tolerate, as the second patient who pulls it out within five minutes demonstrates. The nurses are also concerned that the tube passes through the oesophagus into the stomach and not through the trachea, into the lungs. A coughing and choking patient makes this procedure almost impossible to perform. Nurses are taught to explain what they are doing, how it might feel, and to encourage the patient to swallow by sipping cold water. This helps ease the need to regurgitate and ensures the tube passes into the stomach and not the lungs. They offer constant reassurance throughout. This is the 'rigmarole' Kate refers to. Thus, Kate can go to a senior nurse and check that she has the procedure and 'rigmarole' right. The process of managing the patient's anxiety is built into the procedure and taught as part of it. This is true of the majority of clinical skills, making its inclusion an expectation. The majority of all clinical procedures (from dressings to injections) elicit anxiety: thus the nurse sets out to help the patient manage the body's physical response to this and aid her accomplishment of the task.

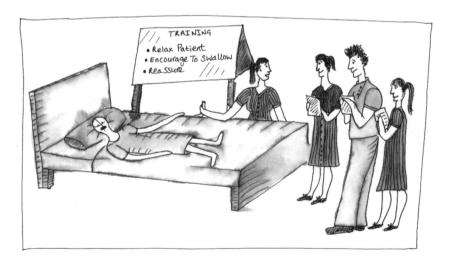

'Learning clinical skills'

Growth in the relationship between the nurse and the patient also occurs. This is because, as in TEL, the processes involved in IEL are informed by feeling rules. The patient is predisposed to trust the nurse's clinical knowledge and expertise, and in their understanding that having a thick latex tube inserted into your mouth, down your throat and into your stomach is not a pleasant experience. The patient trusts the care and expertise of the nurse because he believes she is acting on knowledge that will help preserve and promote his physical wellbeing. While the patient's exclamation, 'Cor that was easy! . . . you must have done hundreds of these', expresses his relief that the procedure is over, it is also an expression of affirmation that his confidence in her competence and expertise to carry out the procedure in a way that minimises his discomfort was met.

The link with the nurse's own development and personality is also different from that of TEL, as seen from the example of the second patient who pulls the tube out. Neither the success in inserting it, nor the apparent overall failure of the task is something that Kate considers important. Kate's inner dialogue illustrates this. She is unconcerned when the patient pulls the tube out. She does not see this as a reflection on her skill. Her emotional labour was instrumental to the action of passing the NG tube in the first instance. This she did successfully. That the patient cannot tolerate it is unconnected to her ability. Rather than re-pass the NG tube, she now sees her role as representing the patient's discomfort to the doctor. In addition, she evaluates the significance of the patient taking out his NG tube in respect to her entire workload. Her inner dialogue reflexively analyses the situation:

> experience tells *me* (her overall identity) that I (here and now in the present) can't force the patient to tolerate the tube, therefore, it is not realistic for *me* to be responsible for the patient not having one. *I* shall get on with the next task, as *I* have lots to do, and if the doctor asks *you* (in the future) why I haven't done it, I'll tell him to do it himself.

She weighs up the overall cost to herself: a single incident of emotional labour undertaken as part of a clinical task is only a part of her responsibilities. Assessing all of her work, her resources and available time, in relation to what she sees as important to her identity, she decides to move on to the next job. Her subject–subject knowledge suggests that the greatest cost of not redoing the tube will come from the doctors. Nurses seldom attribute compassion to doctors (MacKay 1989, 1996; Walby and Greenwell 1994); Kate implies that the doctors might have requested the NG tube as a routine measure rather than as specific to this patient's needs. The doctor does not have to consider the effect it will have on the patient, because the nurse carries out the procedure. Therefore, if the doctor is asked to do it, the doctor may decide that it is not strictly necessary. If it is necessary, the patient is more likely to be reassured by the doctor, as patients place more trust and confidence in doctors' knowledge than in nurses' because of their higher status. In addition, Kate's comment is almost a reflex: '*if* you want it, put it down *yourself*!' reflecting a typically contentious nurse–doctor relationship (MacKay 1989).

When questioned further about her feelings in respect to the task, Kate suggests that it is the accumulation of knowledge and skills that elicits satisfaction. This increases incrementally. Satisfaction elicited from the practical order becomes embedded in the pre-conscious and is linked to performative skills that become pre-reflexive and habitual. Thus Kate draws on these feelings as she brings more and more of her skills together when accomplishing her overall workload, increasingly able to act out her social identity as an efficient competent practitioner. Thus, she states that she feels satisfied at the end of a shift knowing that she has got as much done as possible. Her evaluation of this also reflects the Ward B feeling rule (and is possibly applicable to other areas in nursing) that the amount of work accomplished reflects the degree and skill of the good nurse.

Possibilities

The context for Kate's two stories is set within the boundaries of the outside story: the relationship between the art and science of nursing. Kate refers here to Florence Nightingale, who saw nursing as both an art and a science. She specifically describes the two inside stories in order to explain how the art of nursing (communication skills) is related to the science (clinical skill and knowledge). The ability to relax the patient mentally in order to relax them physically is so important that Kate suggests that she was not able to develop her clinical skills effectively until she had become accomplished in the art of communication.

The value of IEL is well recognised; it is unlikely that any nurse would deny this. However, IEL that is carried out as an integral component of clinical nursing is seldom identified in the literature. As Bone (2002) notes, when emotional labour is being successfully accomplished, it is often hidden from sight. It is hidden for three reasons. First, to nurses, it is largely common sense, an aspect of carrying out clinical skills that has become wholly embedded within the procedure. Second, because it is linked to emotions that are largely pre-reflexive among qualified and experienced nurses, they do not think to mention it. Third, because IEL is taught and monitored, and because it is not considered separate from clinical skills, it is connected to the science of nursing. Equally, the nurse who does not carry out IEL would at best be considered unkind, and at worst, sadistic. These reasons are why Paris does not mention IEL in respect to the clinical side of her work in Vignette 1, 'Half measures'. Rather, she sees emotional labour as being therapeutic and distinct from nurses' clinical roles. It is largely TEL that has become marginalised, compromised due to changes and developments within the profession.

TEL is contentious because it is linked to the Nightingale Ethic and the art of nursing. Salvage (1985), James (1989, 1992), Smith (1992), Witz (1992), Davies (1995) and Philips (1996) argue that the Nightingale Ethic is detrimental to nursing. This is because culturally, it has become connected to nurses' 'natural and inherently feminine' qualities (Smith 1992). Because such qualities are considered intrinsic, and are therefore not required to be taught, they are implicated in the profession's struggle for autonomy. Some also argue that the Nightingale Ethic is detrimental to nursing because it has become synonymous with nurses as self-sacrificial, uncomplaining and submissive (Salvage 1985). In addition, with increasing availability of counsellors, psychotherapists and other allied health care professionals, there is an argument that nurses who are pushed for time should not be taking on roles that can be covered by others.

Although emotional labour is currently conceived as representative of the Nightingale Ethic, in which emotional, psychological care is considered intuitive and separate from the clinical, this is not what Nightingale herself would have advocated. In *Notes on Nursing: What it is and what it is not*, Nightingale wrote: 'It has been said and written a score of times, that every woman makes a good nurse. I believe on the contrary, that the very elements of nursing are all but unknown' (1980 [1859]: 2). Nightingale believed that the essence of nursing 'is to put the patient in the best condition for nature to act upon him' (1980: 110). In order for this to happen she claimed that nursing, as both an art and a science, needed to be both taught and learnt. She emphatically denied that nursing was intuitive to women:

> The everyday management of a large ward, let alone a hospital – the knowing what are the laws of life and death for men, and what are the laws of health for wards (and wards are healthy or unhealthy according to the knowledge or ignorance of the nurse) – are not these matters of sufficient importance and difficulty to require learning by experience and careful inquiry, just as much as any other art? They do not come by inspiration to the lady.
>
> (Nightingale 1980: 111)

Nightingale never intended the 'art and science' of nursing to be separated; nursing care is a combination of both. One of the difficulties with TEL is that it has become separated from the 'science' of nursing, and is no longer considered to be integral to the nursing role. IEL on the other hand is integrated and reveals a different picture about emotional labour in nursing, from which some lessons can be drawn.

Autonomy and investment of self in instrumental emotional labour

Kate makes two significant points about the nature of IEL in respect to her autonomy. The first is that *learning* how and why nurses do what they do is essential to how they manage their emotions. The second is that each microact of IEL and clinical skill contributes towards an overall identity as a competent nurse, which includes the importance of TEL. These points are connected.

Kate believes that managing her emotions in IEL is connected to the learning process. Learning is incremental. Space and time is given to it. Kate notes that:

> I do something new, do it once, twice and again and feel confident and I log it away. And it all gets filed and I suppose you just increase your skill mix don't you as you are learning more and more things and that should be happening all the time and you should be learning something everyday.

This is an attitude, an approach towards personal development. In the context of clinical skills this is one of ongoing forward progression. Kate takes control of her learning and invests in it.

The same attitude is not evident with TEL and its accompanying interpersonal communication skills. Part of the reason for this, noted in Chapter 7, is that nurses often feel defensive about it. There is also a subtle implication within the profession that either nurses are good communicators or they are not. When Kate suggests at the beginning of Vignette 8 that until one has learnt how to behave with people clinical skills cannot be developed, she implies that learning how to behave with people is not an ongoing process. I recently met this attitude in a consultant nurse gynaecology specialist. In an interview researching masters' level work-based learning, she commented that interpersonal communication skills were something one learnt as a student nurse; they are not a masters' level skill. If nurses have not learnt them by a certain point, then they never will. This attitude is prevalent within the profession. Arguably it is because such skills are still connected with the idea that nurses are 'born' to nurse and either are or are not good with people. Having the space and time in which to develop and foster TEL skills is necessary and as Peplau (1988) points out, involves learning about oneself. Investing the self, as a continuous ongoing development of interpersonal communication skills as Kate demonstrates in IEL, is also necessary to TEL.

The link between IEL and identity is also important to why nurses invest themselves in acquiring these skills. For example, in Maxine's interview, she described having sutures removed when she was a young girl:

I had an operation myself. I had a thyroid cyst. I was so impressed. I had sutures in, and of course I had to have them out. And this nurse was doing it for me. I can remember to this day, she just made me feel so relaxed you know. She was talking to me while she was doing it and before I knew it they were out and she goes, 'Well done!' and I said, 'Well done I didn't even feel anything!' and she said, 'Well that is how it should be!' And I can remember her and it is just this real ease that she gave me and this feeling of security and everything.

Maxine told this story in response to a question about what motivated her to become a nurse. Maxine admired the nurse who took out her sutures because of her technical competence and her ease of manner. Much is written about whether or not nurses are 'predisposed' to become nurses because they want to 'care' for people. In this context, 'care' is assumed to relate to women's inherently feminine nature. Yet there is much literature to suggest that care also encompasses practical qualities (Graham 1983; James 1989, 1992). Thus, many nurses note that the reason they want to become nurses is because it is a practical job: caring is helping by doing. Kate notes that she enjoys nursing because:

I like working with people, I'm not one for sitting in an office; it would drive me mad. I like variety, I like being almost independent in what I'm doing. I like being able to work as an independent person. I find people quite interesting. It's not because I want to help people, because I don't, I just want people to be. I don't like people suffering. I don't like people being in pain. I think people suffer quite a lot when they go into hospital for even a minor thing and I just try and put a bit of normality back into it. That's where I come from when I'm at work.

It is because care includes the combination of clinical, hands-on care and emotional labour that nurses find it satisfying (Adams et al. 1998; McNeese-Smith 1999). Similarly, in Vignette 8, Kate states that it is meeting the *challenge* of combining and bringing together all aspects of nursing care – its knowledge, skill, emotional labour, communication and the overall success in the prioritisation and accomplishment of all her workload – that makes her satisfied. This is the import of Kate's final statement in Vignette 8. Thus, for Kate, nursing is both art and science.

The nature of instrumental emotional labour in nursing

The distinction being made between instrumental and TEL is a fine one. The differences in their characteristics are important however, because they reveal different aspects of emotional labour in nursing. The *intention* of IEL is to promote the health and wellbeing of the patient's physical body *by* creating a psychological feeling of security. IEL relaxes the patient psychologically by diverting their attention away from the object of their concern. It is necessary to getting the job done. The successful accomplishment of the task is immediate. Thus, while IEL itself is hidden within the task, its outcome is visible. In contrast the *intention* of TEL is to promote psychological growth and development. It does so *by* encouraging the patient to talk about their feelings. Of course, this can also promote physical wellbeing, although in TEL this is not usually its only intent. TEL deliberately encourages the patient to talk about the reasons for their feelings or concerns. While the need for TEL is obvious, because its purpose is to promote the patient's personal growth and development, the outcome of the labour may not be immediate. It is likely to be part of an ongoing adjustment for the patient. Microacts of TEL contribute towards a more continuous whole, the outcome of which cannot be determined. This is a significant difference, especially since nurses are no longer involved in their patient's entire care trajectory. Many other health care professionals contribute towards an integrated care pathway for patients.

Smith (1992), Davies (1995) and Philips (1996) argue that the marginalisation of emotional labour (by which they mean TEL) has led to a decrease in nurses' satisfaction with their work. It would seem that some of the reason for this is because the way in which TEL is integrated within nursing care has become confused and fragmented. Hilary Graham (1983: 13–14) points out that 'care' encompasses elements of both 'love and labour, identity and activity, with the nature of its demands being shaped by the social relations of the wider society'. Vignettes 1, 2, 5 and 7 all demonstrate that TEL is still an important component of nursing care, that it is still central to the nursing identity and that society – in the form of those nurses care for – still needs and believes in it. While the demands being shaped by the social relations focusing on consumer rights are impacting negatively, the onus is still on the nursing profession to identify how it can carry out effective TEL in twenty-first-century nursing.

Kate's evaluation of the significance of her IEL offers an insight into how this might be accomplished. As noted before, she was not concerned with each individual incidence of IEL; she evaluated it in the context of all her work. This is because of the integrated nature of IEL and the way in which it is linked to identity. Reconceptualising TEL as an integral component of nursing care is necessary, for it is not distinct from nursing's other functions. However, this reconceptualisation needs to recognise that nurses seldom have extended time to spend with their patients, to accept that nurses infrequently carry out hands-on care, and to understand that nursing input into the patient's overall care is fragmented and transitory. Having accepted this, it may be possible to look at how TEL can be reincorporated into nursing care today.

Equally, the emotions connected to IEL are concerned with performative achievement. As noted in Chapter 5, this is a more objective process. In the case of IEL, the nurse either is or is not good at what she does. By the time most nurses qualify, they are moderately self-assured in their clinical skills. Any who have not achieved competency are considered unsafe to practise and are unlikely to be admitted to the Nursing Register. This is an area of nursing care in which they feel assured and confident. In addition, medical development and advancement (DoH 2000), and significant financial and educational investment have been made in this area of nursing. This is not the case with the interpersonal skills necessary to TEL where the personal maturity of the nurse is more relevant. This is more difficult to assess and infinitely more subjective. In addition, the emotions connected to TEL are concerned with self-worth and others' opinions are more involved in their evaluation. This makes the nurse more vulnerable to others. Understanding the process of emotion management is important to identifying how nurses can be facilitated in developing this aspect of their identity. This is explored in more detail in Chapter 9.

Vignette 9 'Breaking the shame spiral'

Kate: I've just done two long days. I was as miserable as sin, basically because of the people I was working with. I cannot work a whole day with some people and if it hadn't have been for them, being immature, loud, being stupid around the desk, I just, I can't work in those conditions. So basically I just shut down and ignored them totally, for maybe the last two-thirds of my day shift. Not a very good way of working. Maybe I'm the one with the problem, I don't know. But I don't like working with immature people. Anyway, for this session, I'm going to cover two subjects, one is the handover from the night shift, and the other one is students.

On the first morning of my first long day, I took over from the night shift. The night staff had basically found a lady who looked like she was going off at 6 o'clock when they did her temperature and blood pressure and she was still quite poorly when I took over. The handover was very, very quick, it took the staff nurse about quarter of an hour to hand over the whole lot, and to get the details about what had gone on with this lady, basically her blood pressure was low, all the things that go with somebody looking as if they're dying. But with regards to the handover I had two HCAs who decided to argue during hand-over about who was going to be doing the breakfast because the ward meeting had said that one HCA from C, D and E bay should do it if there are four, and they then decided to have a ruck about that, and that then carried on for the rest of the morning. The little HCA, who has a very large mouth, carried on in the same strain for the rest of the day, but during the handover, she kept interrupting it in order to tell the staff nurse to hurry up, she hasn't got that sort of time, she needs to get back out on with her patients, this is the HCA speaking by the way, and I knew that I was in for a bad day. And HCAs, as far as I'm concerned, do a bloody fine job, but when it comes to handovers they need to shut their mouths unless there is something concrete that they can add or take away as with the patient care. To start arguing about who is going to be doing breakfast during handover is just bad, bad, bad news.

The second subject that I am going into is that about students. I was able to work with a mature student, Liz, who is a very good nurse. She was my mentor when I worked on rehab, when she was an EN [enrolled nurse: Liz is currently studying to convert from EN to RGN]. She worked very well with me and I feel that she deserves more than what she's been getting on the ward. I feel that she has been very, very let down on the ward, and I think when she has been working with certain people, particularly some staff nurses, they have ignored her and I have witnessed this. They haven't even given her a job to do, or even acknowledged that she is on the ward and I think that that is such bad manners. Anyway, with this particular student, just by sheer coincidence really, because we had this lady who wasn't well in the morning, so they [doctors] wanted an ECG [echo-cardio-gram] done immediately for her. So we went and got the ECG machine from the next door ward and Liz said, 'I've never used one of these machines before, I don't know how to use them'. So I did the ECG and showed her how to use it. And then some minutes later the anaesthetist came on, and literally as he was going through the notes, he said, 'I don't like this ECG, I don't like that one; I want them all done again.' This was for all our pre-op patients basically, I had three patients going to theatres in A bay and every single one had to have their ECGs done. So off our student went and got the ECG machine again and I did the first one with her, with her assisting and let her do the second one, she did it fine and she did the third one on her own. And she was quite competent with doing ECGs. I think it was because she was able to get them done in a very short space of time. And then yesterday I noticed that she was just doing them as a matter of course. I think that that is the best way to learn. Learn about it, do it, do it, so that you have it imprinted in your head. I think that she feels that she was quite happy with that learning experience anyway. When it came to looking at her outcomes, I feel really quite sorry for her because of the fact that she tried to ask me yesterday to look at them. Basically her mentor hasn't been around, and I feel that this lady has been very, very let down indeed. I say it again; I think the ward has let her down big time. And I will get in touch with her today to say that if she can't get her outcomes done, then I'll sign them, 'cos she has worked very, very hard and I have never had a problem with her, although I think that there are some people who have.

Basically on the second day, I had my trimester nine student who is about to qualify. I have mentioned him previously; I decided that he was going to take more responsibility. I let him look after an orthopaedic patient who had suffered a crush injury and I basically advised him that we needed to do all the obs for compartment syndrome and we also kept a very close eye on his other obs because he was quite shocked by what had happened to him. I allowed the student to take him to theatre, to sort him out, and to get him back and he took the care over completely. So he knew about this patient when it come to handover. He didn't want to do the handover in the evening . . . I was going to go home, because I really wasn't feeling very good, I was totally miserable about being at work and I just wanted to go home and I did ask if I could take some time owing to me, but I decided against it because I felt that I needed to be with my student to hand over and coach him through it and give him more encouragement, because of the way he has been and because he has been let down by myself as well, because I am still learning how to be a mentor and I do take that role seriously and I will continue to do so. Basically I coached him through the handover before we did the handover. I suggested he keep his bit of paper as well so that he could say anything that he had written down over the day and all the obs and things we were doing; and I explained to him the rationale behind saying what type of nutritional status somebody was at. And we went in and I just looked at him and he went ahead. I came out thinking that he had done quite well. He said to me that he felt that he was much more structured and he knew where he was going now-on-in in handover, so basically we're going to practise that from now onwards. And that will be much better for him really.

There. That's my positive attitude point of my second long day of this week. But other than that I could quite happily have left yesterday, because I am not part of the crowd that are there and I most of all don't wish to be part of it. I don't find it very nice; I don't find it very professional. I don't find it professional sitting on the nurses' station trying to get the loudest fart to ripple along and to make the loudest noises. If anybody did that in a shop they would be sacked. Because it's a hospital these people think that they can get away with it and I think that it is disgusting.

This is me after night duty. I didn't realise how upset I was about the people I have been working with. Because quite out of the blue in the middle of handover, we were just generally chatting about the way people behave on the ward and I just burst out crying. I thought I was angry, I didn't know I was that upset. I really thought I was more angry than upset. And basically somebody told Daisy, so she knew and she had to deal with it. Last night, she was going to go home, I think, and all of a sudden she didn't, she just come back and said to me, 'Kate, I need to know what it's all about'. And I told her how I felt. And I think she knows that this is going on. Apparently I was the fourth person in one day to complain about these particular people's behaviour and I feel better now that I've spoken about it. I also feel better because I know that I'm not a crap nurse after all the digs and the jibes and the checking up on me and basically doing things that undermine my confidence. I know I'm not crap, I know I'm not because I've dealt with every shift this week I have dealt with a crisis situation and I did it again last night on my own, and without a doctor for a good hour and a half of the crisis, because although I was bleeping him, he was held up. The hospital was humming last night. There was admissions and emergencies everywhere. We had four admissions while I also had this lady who was being unwell and what I can't believe, is this lady had been left not cared for properly because she had had a CVA [cerebral vascular accident] . . . [Double recorded] . . . I can't believe that she had been left all day with her 2.5 and 2.8 2.9 BMs [blood glucose/sugar levels]. Why are people doing her BMs and ignoring it? Nobody did anything about her BMs apart from put 5% glucose through her system on a drip [1000mls over eight hours]. I took it into my own hands and I phoned up site sister and basically got permission to give her glucose [10% in 10mls, statutory dose] on a verbal order and once the doctor came up he realised that the situation wasn't too good and we went all out to help her in the end. My main concern was that she was dying in pain 'cos she was very, very alert and in a great deal of pain and none of us could really put it down as to what it was. The handover wasn't too bad, and I'll tell you for why. It was because I did a handover with two mature nurses and two mature HCAs who were working towards getting as much information about their patients rather than trying to talk about their social life. Anyway that was that then.

This is the day after quite a good shift actually. I enjoyed the people I was working with and I enjoyed the work I did and I felt quite good about it. I had a good day yesterday as I said because I didn't have any crises and I wasn't working on my own, I got my work done and also I liked the people I was working with. So, that makes a lot of difference.

This will be my last report. I feel that I have turned a corner at work. Maybe I've had a ward to shed, maybe my blowout has helped me. But the most positive thing I have realised in the last week to ten days is that I can do my job. And a little while ago I doubted myself, I wasn't sure that I could do it. I think that it was because I was feeling less confident myself for obvious reasons already mentioned before this, and I know I can do this job because I have been doing it and I do, do it and I know that I am not perfect and I'm a human being and I have times when some days I do the job better than others depending on how I feel.

9   Collegial emotional labour

This chapter looks at collegial emotional labour, which relates to the relationships nurses have with each other and within the multidisciplinary team. Because it is not directly concerned with patients or their relatives, its character is different from that of therapeutic and instrumental emotional labour. Personal differences between colleagues are more significant in collegial emotional labour because issues of status and place are more fluid. Thus, the link between emotional labour and personal identity is more apparent. This chapter analyses the nature of Kate's collegial emotional labour described in Vignette 9. The vignette, taken from the second half of her audio diary, documents Kate's personal feelings over ten days. It provides a unique opportunity to examine her inner dialogue and explore how personal and social identity are intertwined and expressed through her collegial emotional labour. From this, authenticity of self in emotional labour is evaluated.

Collegial emotional labour

Effective communication is essential to everyday nursing practice. Patients and their relatives, however, are not the only people with whom nurses interact and develop relationships. Nurses work with one another, HCAs, students, doctors, ward clerks, occupational therapists, physiotherapists, social workers, theatre staff, pharmacists, managers, porters, domestic staff, agency staff and many others. Only the nurses are fixed and constant to the ward; most other health care professionals come and go. As such, nurses act as communication conduits through whom important information is presented, processed and passed on. The hectic pace and huge quantity of their work significantly impacts on this, as do inevitable conflicts between people. Nurses' collegial emotional labour (CEL) is therefore vital to this process, especially as communication can go awry. This might be because information is passed on when the nurse is in the middle of doing something else; or because miscommunication occurs between professionals; or because there is a personal conflict between them or a difference of opinion over the best way to manage patient care.

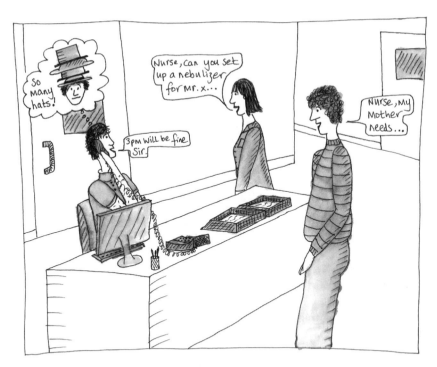

'Communication conduit'

Emily: Handover took approximately 25 minutes, um there were two outside interruptions. One was a HCA coming in to say she had given a diabetic a cake and she felt really bad about it, so we spent a few minutes talking to her and telling her that it didn't matter really because at the end of the day, the person was hypo anyway. And another interruption was another HCA coming in to let me know there would be an admission from HDU [High Dependency Unit] during the night and telling me what the patient was and that we needed to move a couple of beds round for that.

Maria: The pharmacist made me very angry. He didn't pick a few things out so I had to do requests for certain treatment cards in the afternoon. I had no help from physios as well. I asked them to come back before lunchtime to take patient out from bed to chair by hoist as he was very heavy. He just had stroke so I didn't feel confident to do it on my own. And they didn't come back and the patient was very upset and his wife was very upset and I had to apologise to them.

Amelia: The doctors came round were just totally out of order, totally arrogant towards the nursing staff, wanting to know why things hadn't been done when they hadn't even been asked for. And when I told them about the chap in rm. 3 [Alix from Vignette 2], pulling his NG tube out at least every four hours and having to be re-sited every four hours for his feeds, they thought this was a huge joke. Well they commentated that we could get a lot of practice that way and I said that it wasn't me that needed the practice, it was the doctors, which was even funnier from their point of view. And when I asked them about a peg [a permanent tube inserted directly into the stomach for feeding], they said there was no way they could do a peg at weekends so this poor chap has to be tortured every four hours so that we can get his medication and his feeds down him. And I just feel that that is just totally unacceptable.

CEL is also necessary when conversing with colleagues in the presence of patients and relatives. For example, when caring for a woman with massive haemorrhaging, it was necessary to advise a newly qualified doctor that he needed to organise an emergency theatre for the patient without damaging the patient's confidence in him. Communication with other members of the ward team can sometimes be fraught with conflict due to clashes in personality, or as a result of bullying, as is evident in Vignette 9. Such variants are implicated in the nature of CEL.

'Collegial' is a term which comes from the Latin word *collega* meaning pertaining to one's colleague's (Readers Digest 1993: 277) and involving shared responsiblity (*Concise Oxford Dictionary* 1999). The purpose of CEL is to promote effective communication between the nurse and her colleagues in order to facilitate nursing care. The feeling rules related to CEL are primarily associated with mediating everyday courtesy and manners as well as interprofessional health care issues; they are fluid and more nebulous in nature than those pertaining to TEL or IEL. This is for several reasons. First, this aspect of emotional labour is less regulated and monitored. The 'meanings and values are not stable and fixed but are in a constant process of change and modification' (Burkitt 2002: 153). The outcome in CEL is not necessarily predictable; rather it is negotiable because there is not necessarily a 'correct' result to the interaction. In the quotation above for example, Emily carries out CEL with the HCA who has mistakenly given a patient with diabetes a cake. The patient in question is fortunately hypoglycaemic at the time. Thus, Emily reassures the HCA, who is very penitent. This interaction might have had a different outcome if the patient had not been hypoglycaemic.

Second, CEL is more ambiguous in its outcome, because its purpose is not as defined within constraining social values and norms as TEL and IEL are. For example, in the quotation above, Amelia presents her perspective of a situation concerning a patient for whom she is concerned; the doctor's perspective, however, is different. They need to negotiate and compromise in order to ensure that the patient's best interests are met. CEL is important within such exchanges. The connection between feeling rules and image in CEL is also more fluid. For example, the relationship between doctors and

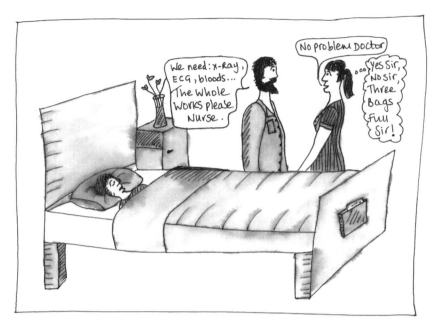

'The handmaiden!'

nurses is typically contentious, and has a long history (Mackay 1989, 1993, 1996; Walby and Greenwell 1994). However, their relationship is continuously evolving, whereas the interdependent nature of medicine and nursing remains constant. Feeling rules concerned with their relationship reflect this. Thus, in the example with Amelia, the contentious relationship between doctors and nurses is more evident. However, in Vignette 9, Kate and the doctor interact harmoniously as they work together in caring for the patient with a CVA.

Third, the variable in CEL may not be the outcome but the person. In Vignette 9, Kate responds very differently to individual nurses and HCAs. This is to do with personality. Thus, while the interaction might be carried out as part of the nurse's role, it is not necessarily constrained by social norms and values pertaining to that role. CEL is directly associated with the individuals because how an individual carries out their emotion management in these situations is representative of characteristics related to their personal identity.

All these characteristics are present in TEL and IEL. However, the feeling rules feel more nebulous and fluid in CEL because of differences in place and status between colleagues. These can be varied due to the individual's professional role, or because of individual personality differences. Although personal identity is also embedded within TEL and IEL, interaction between nurse and the patient or relative is mediated by their social identity where the nurse has a higher status and therefore greater power (see Figure 9.1, page 196). Thus it is understood that the nurse manages her emotions for the patient's benefit. CEL is more fluid because status between health care professionals is less defined and fluctuates. It can be used therefore as a status marker. Because of this, sometimes the person with a lower status has to manage their emotions while those with a higher one are free to express theirs.

Thus, while CEL is related to general feeling rules within the work environment, it is also regulated by feeling rules, attitudes, norms and values specific to a *particular* workplace. 'Collegial' is also related to the French word *collège*, taken from the Latin *collegium* (Readers Digest 1993: 227). In addition to referring to one's colleagues therefore, collegial also relates to the idea of a college, an institution known for its particular traditions, attitudes, values and norms. On Ward B, for example, many of the ward's norms and feeling rules were related to issues of bullying, subgroup identity and power struggles (see Chapter 6). These issues are specific to that ward, but other wards, or workplaces, such as a sociology department, a local church or mosque or branch of a national bank would also have their own particular sets of values, attitudes and feeling rules. CEL therefore manages emotions that arise from the social order. They are concerned with self-worth and the expression of personal and social identity especially in respect to place and status; for it is in the workplace that individuals express their sense of self while carrying out their duties and working with their colleagues (see Table 9.1).

Collegial emotional labour in 'Breaking the shame spiral' (Vignette 9)

Kate had been experiencing bullying for several months prior to recording her audio diary. Vignette 9 illustrates how CEL can represent place and status

Table 9.1 Collegial emotional labour

Purpose	Emotions	Skills	Feeling rules
To facilitate effective communication between colleagues in order to promote effective nursing care.	Subject–subject emotions concerned with self-worth and personal and social identity.	Interpersonal communication skills.	Are concerned with general courtesy and manners.
To assert status rights over one's colleagues.			Are concerned with professional identity and role.
To acknowledge one's place in respect to one's colleagues.			Are local to specific workplaces.

and demonstrates how it can be used to challenge that place. Her inner dialogue also reveals the intertwining of her personal and social identity in the articulation and rearticulation of her feelings through the passage of four important stories. In Kate's interview some months later, from which some excerpts below are included, this process can be seen to have been consolidated.

Boundaries

Vignette 9 has three distinct but related emotional communiqués (Sandelands and Boudens 2000). There is the overt communiqué in which Kate moves from having no status to establishing both status and place on the ward. Thus, in itself, the diary could be said to be status marker. There is the communiqué in which Kate reasserts her sense of personal identity through her renegotiated social identity as a member of Ward B. However, the primary communiqué is Kate's management of unacknowledged shame, which is hidden within the other two communiqués.

Kate's emotions mostly emerge from the social order and are concerned with self-worth. Initially she battles *unacknowledged* shame, elicited as a result of bullying. In the interview Kate confesses that the other nurses 'were condescending and just implying that I wasn't doing my job properly um, sideways, bang on, head on, they were at it all the time'. In the diary the shame is unacknowledged until Kate has her 'blowout' after which she admits that she had doubted her abilities. Unacknowledged shame can become reactive with other emotions, such as anger, in a cycle of emotion, which continually responds to it, creating shame–anger spirals (Lewis 1971). For example, Kate might feel humiliated and shamed at the suggestion of being incompetent, and then immediately feel angry at the suggestion of incompetence; she might then feel ashamed of feeling angry at those who suggest she is incompetent; then feel anger towards herself, in a continuous spiral of shame–anger–shame–anger. Lewis (1971) also called this 'humiliated fury'. Emotions of anger, doubt, disgust and anxiety linked to shame (Lewis 1971; Kemper 1978, 1990; Scheff 1990; Katz 1999; Barbalet 2002) certainly dominate Kate's diary. However, throughout the text it is surges of anger that seep through in mini-tirades concerning the staff nurses' behaviour; the HCAs interrupting handover; the bad mentoring of the students; and the poor care of the CVA patient. After her outburst, Kate admits that she was feeling angry but was unaware of feeling so upset about it all. This suggests that Kate's CEL focused on suppressing feelings of anger. This suppression, however, was frequently unsuccessful because the anger was really a result of unacknowledged shame due to bullying.

In addition to suppressing anger, Kate was also inducing it. For example, her anger motivated her to isolate herself and was influential in her developing disgust at the behaviour of her colleagues. This is indicative of deep emotion management: Kate needs to believe that she is angry rather than ashamed. Drawing on Freud (see Chapter 4), it is possible to see that Kate induces anger and consciously interprets her repressed shame as anger. Her anger, therefore, is the 'ideational presentation' of repressed shame. Consequently, her feelings of shame are neither consciously suppressed, nor unconsciously repressed. Her anger is no less authentic for being induced. However, the unacknowledged shame contributes towards the shame–anger spiral in which she is caught up, making the anger volatile. Thus, Kate repeatedly expresses anger at situations that relate to her feelings of inadequacy and shame, and resulting ultimately in her precipitous breakdown.

The vignette begins with a statement of how miserable she is; that she cannot work with certain people so she has shut down, but maybe she is the one with the problem. She does not know. Kate acknowledges her anxiety and feelings of inadequacy, expressing a lack of confidence and a sense of isolation from the other nurses. Shame can result in feelings related to a lack of security and are usually the ones individuals admit to (Lewis 1971; Scheff 1990; Katz 1999; Barbalet 2001). Kate's repression of her shame and her suppression of anxiety, anger and loss of confidence impact on her sense of personal identity and in her acts of CEL express her social identity. Thus her CEL demonstrates her low status on the ward.

'As long as it persists, shame carries the sense that there is revealed an undeniable truth about the self. The matters that one is ashamed about are acknowledged as fundamental to one's character' (Katz 1999: 150). In order to re-establish her personal identity Kate needs to overcome the bullying and the shame it has elicited, and challenge the place the others have given her. Not to do this would be to accept the other nurses' assessment of her as an 'undeniable truth'. This had previously been the case in the preceding two and half months.

> Constructing a sense of one's relative place involves self-evaluation and comparison, and these activities evoke feelings of, for example, pain, shame and belittlement or pride, pleasure and empowerment. Sending a place message can evoke some of these feelings in the other. The emotion conveys information about the state of the social ranking system: it informs us where we stand and tells others where they do or should stand.
>
> (Clark 1990: 308)

Initially, it is the other nurses who send place messages, but Kate challenges this when she confesses to the G grade sister. She achieves this change through a series of different expressions of identity, as they grow and develop in actions of performance, identification and belonging. Through the course of her inner dialogue, her shame and anger dissipate, and disgust and indignation emerge as second order emotions. The dialogic process occurs through four recognisable stories within the whole extract that are integral to the overall narrative. The first is concerned with the unprofessional behaviour of the other staff nurses. This is the overriding story that changes tenor and punctuates the other three: the HCAs' bad behaviour during handover, the students and being a mentor, and nursing the woman with a CVA. Through these stories Kate works towards a stronger assertion of self. Satisfaction and pride emerge and become more significant as she re-evaluates her nursing abilities and place in the ward's hierarchy. She describes the process as having 'a ward to shed'. The intertwining of Kate's personal and social identity emerges through this process.

Dynamic tensions

The dynamic tensions are set out within the four stories. In the first two, Kate depicts the HCAs and the nurses asserting their privileges of elevated place.

> Those occupying higher place have more esteem and privilege. They have more and different interactional rights, including the right to evaluate others, ask personal questions, give advice, point out flaws, have their opinions count, be late, have something more important to do, ignore the other and so on.
>
> (Clark 1990: 306)

Kate's decision to accept or deny the behaviour of the other nurses trying to impose their interactional rights is the primary dynamic. Within this dynamic Kate defines and redefines who the insiders and the outsiders are, re-evaluating her own place.

In the interview Kate describes the behaviour of the other staff in more detail:

> Well this particular day, which I think really sparked me off and kept with me for a few days until I broke down, was the fact that they were all sitting on the nurses' desk, sitting on the desk, not just sitting to the right or to the left, but sitting on the desk farting as loud as they could. And I was round the corner by the doctor's desk and I could hear them. And they were screaming with laughter. It was like they were in a pub. Now, I wouldn't want to be with people in a pub like that, let alone at work. We're professionals who have got uniforms on, who have done training. We are supposed to be putting over a respectful dignified exterior because we have to portray ourselves in a certain way because we are going to tell people what to do with their lives. You don't do that after you have just farted on a table to make it really loud! That is not nice. It just isn't nice it is just not the way to behave. That afternoon they had also locked themselves in the treatment room. They had barricaded it because they were practising venflons on each other [inserting needles into veins]. Unprofessional? Unethical? They hadn't even done the

course. Now to me, that is so wrong, and these people are still on the ward. There was no respect for their patients, and that really peed me off big time because that is my paramount thing.

The other nurses are grouped together either around the nurses' station or barricaded in the treatment room. This excludes Kate and identifies her as the outsider. By barricading themselves into the treatment room to practise venflon insertion, they assert their privileges of elevated place and power; effectively creating an intimacy for those included behind the barricaded doors and distancing those who are excluded on the other side. Part of Kate's CEL is an acceptance of their exclusion of her. Although Kate strenuously identifies their unprofessional behaviour in the interview, her initial response in the diary is more reflective of her exclusion. This is evident when she chooses to tell the story of the students before she explains what their behaviour was, and then she tells only part of it. The revelation that they barricaded themselves into the treatment room to practise venflon insertion comes only in the interview. This is because the act of exclusion is an act of rejection and results in Kate doubting herself at the same time as she is ashamed of their behaviour. Thus, as at the beginning of the diary excerpt, she says: 'Maybe I'm the one with the problem. I don't know'. From this point of doubt, she chooses to tell the story about the HCAs' behaviour in handover.

This story reinforces the dynamic tension of insiders and outsiders. Here the HCAs decide to discuss who is going to do breakfast during handover. The face-to-face status they impose here is impressive. Not only do they displace the official ranking between HCAs and nurses but they do so by elevating their role of giving breakfast to one of more importance than that of caring for the critically ill patient. Kate's emotions here reflect the shame–anger spiral. Ultimately this results in a loss of confidence and anxiety in losing face. Thus, Kate states that this is going to be a bad shift, acknowledging the power the HCAs exert over her. Kate does not document any confrontation with the HCAs over their behaviour, suggesting that in her CEL she suppressed her shame and anger during the shift, expressing them only in her diary.

Through these two stories, Kate acknowledges her place as an outsider and the tensions this elicits in her. But this is Kate's diary, Kate's narrative. As an outsider and in the safe space of the diary, Kate admits her doubts that her competency as a nurse is questionable (an expression of her personal identity). But she also acknowledges that she feels embarrassment at the unprofessional conduct of her colleagues (an expression of her social identity). In putting these two stories together, Kate expresses her doubt concerning her competency and expresses a burgeoning challenge to that doubt, thereby identifying this tension within herself. It is likely, therefore, that Kate's CEL in which she suppressed her feelings of anger and shame was also an act of self-protection.

Her separation from the other ward staff creates a space within the narrative to introduce a new group: the students. The story of the students adds three important dynamics to the overall emotional communiqué. First, Kate identifies herself with the students and their situation; second, in her interaction with them, her social identity as their mentor establishes a positive aspect to her personal identity; third, she builds up a good versus bad nurse discourse.

First, in taking on the role of mentor Kate identifies with the students rather than the other staff nurses. With Liz, there is a prior relationship from when the roles were reversed – Kate being the student and Liz the mentor. Through this bond she implies that her relationship with Liz is based on respect, in contrast to her lack of respect for the other nurses. Kate's projection of her own desire to learn (an aspect of personal identity revealed in Vignette 8) on to Liz indicates that transference is taking place. Kate empathises with her need to learn, and in respect to Liz's previous role, wishes to reciprocate by teaching her well (suggestive of introjective identification of Liz's need). There is also a sense that Kate is projecting her own feelings in her realisation that Liz has been let down by the other nursing staff; as a newly qualified nurse Kate is still learning the ropes, yet she has been given very little support to help her adjust and learn her new responsibilities as a staff nurse. Kate states twice: 'I feel that this lady has been very, very let down indeed. I say it again; I think the ward has let her down big time.' The strength of her empathy reflects an unconscious realisation that she has also been let down ('I-Thou' attitude). Thus, she need not judge herself so harshly because in fact she has managed to adjust to her new role as D grade with little help from the more senior nurses. This transference is an important part of the process of individuation; it enables Kate to perceive her own identity as a newly qualified nurse as being distinct from that of the other more experienced nurses ('I-It' attitude). With the second student she notes that she is also new to mentoring. However, she is no longer a student so it is right for her to take on the role of mentor. Through her transference with the students, Kate accepts that although she is newly qualified and cannot be as competent as more experienced nurses, she has managed very well and has the capacity to act with maturity and responsibility. Thus, the students play an important part in the re-evaluation of her place. The growing dynamic in which she sees herself as a good mentor facilitates the development of the good versus bad nurse dynamic.

By successfully teaching Liz how to do ECGs and the male student how to improve his handover skills, Kate also experiences satisfaction. Liz's success in learning to do ECGs reinforces Kate's perception of the importance of learning by observation, support and practice. Because satisfaction is elicited from the practical order it is perceived as an objective witness to her teaching success. Although Liz is a person (subject–subject relationship), in the action of teaching, Kate objectifies her because the process of teaching is procedural and the result is skill based ('I-It' attitude). Thus, in explaining her aim of teaching Liz to carry out ECGs, Kate goes into detail about how she taught her. Thus, she emphasises her teaching *skills* which have elicited satisfaction and reinforced an important aspect of her personal identity. Now, to a degree, the results of the teaching are independent of Kate's subjective relationship with Liz, in that if she had not successfully taught her how to do an ECG, she quite simply would not be able to do one. Kate, therefore, directly derives emotions of satisfaction in the success of her teaching skills, which within a finite time frame are independent of the social dialogue concerned with the effect of bullying or her subjective relationship with the students. It is arguable that the reason this story – and the success she has in teaching the male student to hand over – is included because she was successful. This suggests that in this instance the emotions of satisfaction elicited from the practical order, are *prior* to subjective feelings of pride because she consciously or unconsciously chooses the story to illustrate her point about being a good mentor based on her success.

Having experienced satisfaction in her ability as a mentor, Kate then derives pride in presenting her social identity as a good mentor versus the other nurses as bad mentors (subject–subject relations). These emotions are very important to her self-worth. At this point Kate suddenly resumes the overriding story about the other nurses, only now the good versus bad nurses dynamic becomes much more apparent. This is where the male student nurse's story is important; for Kate decides to stay at work to coach him through handover despite feeling miserable and unwell. This is in contrast to other mentors who have let him, Liz and ultimately Kate, down. In being a good mentor, Kate experiences pride (social order emotion) in addition to satisfaction (practical order). Her CEL with the students reinforces her sense of personal identity which is performed through her social identity as a mentor (Katz 1999; Archer 2000). Thus, in suppressing her feelings of misery, and encouraging and promoting her student instead, through her CEL Kate acts professionally, beginning the re-establishment of her identity as a 'good nurse'. Thus, she has begun to re-evaluate her personal identity as a good nurse through her social identity as a good mentor. This re-evaluation is not completed however as her comment: 'I am not part of the crowd that are there and I most of all don't wish to be part of it' expresses continuing conflict. However, it is moderated in that she acknowledges her desire to be separate from them.

From these stories, unacknowledged, suppressed or repressed emotions of anger, shame, anxiety, empathy, satisfaction and pride have emerged. The tension they create makes her feel unwell: 'I really wasn't feeling very good'. In the interview she expands on this:

> I felt physically sick before I went into work, I felt very emotional all the time. Very sort of wobbly as well, you know where you feel like you have got butterflies in your stomach all the time. It was like I was the new girl

every single day for about two and half months. I shouldn't be feeling like this! I was questioning myself all the time. But physically I felt sick and it wasn't until I burst out crying in the middle of a handover, which embarrassed me quite a lot, that it actually came to a head. I was getting unhealthy as well. I was getting quite bad skin and my eyes were really dark all the time; I had permanent bags under my eyes. I was sleeping like there was no tomorrow. I was sleeping, sleeping and sleeping, and I was struggling to get up in the morning, which is a sign of depression actually, isn't it, if you don't want to get up and all you want to do is go to sleep? And I was just walking around knackered all the time. And I think that was due to the fact that I was having such a hard time at work.

In effect Kate creates a pressure cooker of unexpressed bottled-up emotions (Lupton 1998), which initially cause her to feel unwell. Then during handover, these emotions suddenly erupt. Following the outburst, Kate comments that she was unaware of how 'upset' she was really feeling. This suggests that her outburst brought a conscious awareness of those feelings. Such emotional outbursts can be 'understood as a means of gaining an insight into the "true" self, for in their very "naturalness" they are perceived as breaking through the bonds of "culture" . . . revealing to oneself how one is really responding to a phenomenon' (Lupton 1998: 89). This seems to be the case with Kate who, following this outburst, acknowledges that the bullying made her feel ashamed and anxious to the degree that she had questioned her abilities. She also comments on how the outburst embarrassed her. Through her 'blowout' Kate also expresses her disgust at the behaviour of her colleagues. This expression brings the realisation that she has been ashamed of them because she is also a member of the ward team. Thus, Kate realises that she has been shamed *by* these nurses in the suggestion that she is a bad nurse; second, she has been ashamed *about* their behaviour; and third, *she* is ashamed that it was this group of nurses who she allowed to bully her. The outburst that Kate experiences when she bursts into tears in front of a *different* group of nurses brings a degree of conscious realisation about this threefold process of shame and is the point at which she breaks the shame–anger spiral. The outburst results in an opportunity for Kate to confess what has been happening to the G grade. In doing so she sends a place marker to the bullies saying she will no longer be intimidated by them. Her outburst represents the culmination of the dynamic tensions.

Growth

When an individual is shamed as Kate has been, they often attempt to redress their shameful action (Barbalet 2001). In the story of the woman with a CVA, there is a sense that it is important that Kate's acts are seen as restitution for her previous embarrassment and humiliation. The other nurses are more obviously 'bad' nurses now, and Kate's nursing care, almost entirely absent from the previous stories, reappears, demonstrating her competency and skill.

Instead of feeling anxious about who she is working with, Kate is anxious about her patient. She is concerned over her low blood sugar levels and her pain. She is also angry on behalf of her patient, who she implies has not received proper care from the staff on the previous shift. These emotions are important. By making the contrast between her care and that of the other nurses, Kate is *motivated to trust* her judgement in implementing appropriate care. The emotions that subsequently emerge reward that trust: satisfaction (practical order) that she took the correct course of action using her own initiative, and pride (social order) that her actions were supported by the site sister and the doctor. As in the story of the students, Kate demonstrates her skill and knowledge by describing how she cares for the stroke patient when she successfully corrects her blood glucose level and reduces her pain. Again, these are competency skills from which her successful performance elicits satisfaction. Her actions are procedural. She draws on both embedded natural and practical skills and discursive knowledge in diagnosing the low blood glucose, identifying the correct treatment, uncovering a policy to support her diagnosis and treatment (when the doctor is unable to attend), carrying out that treatment, and in monitoring the results which show that the blood sugar is raised. Her success produces indisputable knowledge and assurance that she is not incompetent in her nursing skill in the direct subject–object relationship that she has with the patient's physical body. That body cannot 'lie'; it does not give a subjective opinion based on its impression of Kate. It reacts according to scientific and medical principles which Kate can take as true evidence. Thus, when she makes her argument that she is not a 'crap' nurse, she has an objective supporter, reinforced by the satisfaction she feels in response to her task and in the subsequent approval that she gains from others.

Kate's next diary entry reflects the realisation that she can do her job. Once this realisation is achieved, she notices that there are some staff nurses – those in the alpha seniors and the beta group – that she likes working with: a significant fact which she comments on. Kate recognises that she has turned a corner, commenting that she has had 'a ward to shed'. Thus, significant growth has occurred.

Possibilities

New possibilities present themselves on the horizon. Kate acknowledges that she still needs space to learn, but not being perfect does not make her a bad nurse. Thus, the impact of the bullying has successfully been re-evaluated. In her acts of CEL Kate's inner dialogue has passed through the process of discernment, deliberation and dedication (see Chapter 5). First order emotions are identifiable. Kate's 'I' draws on her feelings at present, for example (paraphrasing the central themes and emotions):

> I feel miserable because I have doubted my nursing abilities, I have experienced shame on having qualified but not successfully acting as a good D grade (social). I have lost confidence and experienced dissatisfaction with my clinical skills and knowledge (practical). I have been feeling physically sick from fear and anxiety anticipating a hostile reception at work (natural).

In the *discernment phase* there is awareness that she has a choice to make. Kate appeals to her 'you' in the future from her 'me' in the past:

> Like me, these students are motivated to learn, I am motivated to learn, I invested myself in nursing, I enjoy it and gain satisfaction from it and being a nurse makes me feel proud. Even though I feel miserable at the moment, I can see that I am a good mentor in comparison to the other nurses. However, I am actually a new staff nurse, still learning, therefore I should not judge myself so harshly. You should consider the fact that you are better than you think, for I have successfully managed my nursing care including the lady with a CVA, therefore, I still gain satisfaction and pride in my work.

Her CEL here enables her to identify with the students.

In the *deliberation phase* there is a weighing up of the cost:

> I might not be a member of this particular group of nurses, but I can invest in what I consider to be a nurse. I am not a team member, therefore, I chose to work and act alone. This will cost me esteem in the eyes of the other nurses, but in my own eyes I will be a good nurse again. Is the loss of esteem in the eyes of the other nurses really important to my self-worth and integrity? Perhaps I really am a bad nurse?

Her CEL here allows her to isolate herself from the other nurses, thereby creating valuable space in which she can identify with other aspects of her role.

In the *dedication phase* she sets out to reach an accommodation with these different emotions.

> Because I have separated myself from the others I can see that their behaviour disgusts me. Actually I know that I am a good nurse because of the way I handled the lady with a CVA. As a result of my outburst I can admit that I was really feeling disgust about the other nurses and shame that I have let them bully me. These feelings are more significant than my self doubt.

The cost of isolation is lessened when she receives support from different nurses reinforcing her own assessment: thus second order emotions re-establish her self-worth and identity as a member of Ward B.

Kate can now take the moral high ground. She has voluntarily separated from the group not because they have isolated her, nor because she is a bad nurse but because she is a good nurse and they are not. She has re-established feelings of self-worth, investing again in emotions that elicit pride. By the time of her interview this rationale has fully developed:

> One of the things that I have always stuck with me, while I was training as well, is that I love nursing. Nursing to me deserves a lot of respect because we deal with the shite of life. One way or the other we get the toilet of life, we really do and I feel that if you are going to go to work you should go to work and have a bit of dignity yourself, because how can you portray and how can you give other people dignity if you can't even behave in a dignified manner. I don't believe in shouting your mouth off, just because you are at work and you are on a hospital ward, you shouldn't be sitting around shouting your mouth off. You don't do that, you don't do that in the street. I don't let my children behave like that the way some of those people have been behaving. My children would get slapped and they would be kept in. I take great pride in being a nurse, I am very proud of the fact that I am a nurse and that I have an amount of power. It is, it's power. There is an amount of power, and I take a great deal of pride that I don't abuse that. You know I don't abuse that, and if I start to abuse that, I want out. And I think that these people abuse that power.

Kate's second order emotions centre on socially defined and morally and culturally constituted issues. Through her inner dialogue and CEL she has reinforced her sense of identity and brought personal and social justification. In the extract above, Kate talks about being a mother, acting professionally, with dignity and composure, using emotional labour similar to that which is represented in the Nightingale Ethic: these characteristics are related to the alpha senior subgroup. The growth and movement in the inner dialogue shows how Kate has repudiated the alpha populars' place for her in the beta group, and re-established herself as an alpha senior. Kate has realigned herself, and identified a new place in which she can act out her personal identity as a professional, competent nurse through her social identity as a staff nurse in the alpha seniors. Her CEL now reflects this new place and status on Ward B.

Authenticity and autonomy of self in collegial emotional labour

> Identity is more than self-reflection, understanding and the development of a life-project based on the idea of a calling. It is fundamentally about issues of belonging, expression, performance, identification and communication with others.
>
> (Hetherington 1998: 62)

For Hochschild (1983), the transmutation of private emotion work into public emotional labour ultimately leads to self-inauthenticity due to the suppression of 'real' feelings and the expression of 'false' ones in their place. This implies not only that personal (private) and social (public) identity are always expressed independently of one another, but also that the 'true self' (personal identity) is a fixed, knowable entity that requires constant expression, through readily identifiable 'real' feelings. Kate's CEL suggests that there is a different interpretation. First, it shows that personal and social identity are intertwined. Second, those expressions of personal identity continually grow and develop in response to different aspects of self and to different challenges and experiences met along the way. In Kate, those observable aspects of self are related to her sense of personal identity, her performative and social identity as a nurse and her place in the Ward B team. Third, it shows that the suppression or repression of 'real' feelings does not necessarily equate with the expression of a 'false' self. To suggest they do, devalues the importance of emotional labour to nursing and the integrity and autonomy of the individual carrying it out.

Although personal identity is distinct from social identity, they are intertwined. Archer (2000) suggests that personal identity emerges through the inner dialogue, regulating aspects of self-worth, understandings of material competency and orientating self to the natural (environment and visceral) world.

> Personal identity, which has been seen to result from the subject's considered response to its encounters with nature, practice and society, via the internal conversation, must not be confounded with social identity. Although the two are intertwined, and indeed their emergence will be presented as dialectical process, personal identity is always broader than social identity because it is the former which both animates the latter and defines its standing relative to other concerns, which social concerns do not necessarily outweigh. Social identity is only assumed in society: personal identity regulates the subjects' relations with reality as a whole.
>
> (Archer 2000: 257)

The emotions expressed in Vignette 9 are integral to the orientation of the self towards reality and a sense of self in the emergence of personal identity

– aspects of which emerge through Kate's social identity as a nurse on Ward B. Thus, it is not just Kate's social identity that is affected by the bullying, it is her whole self. Even in the safety of her own home she 'was sleeping like there was no tomorrow' and in the interview confessed that she found it difficult to talk about it to her husband. Kate experienced a variety of emotions over a period of time, reflexively managing them through her internal conversation. During this time, it was necessary for her to go to work and present social identities of nurse, mentor and colleague. Kate's CEL enables her to present these social identities which, because they are understood through, and regulated by her personal identity, are also expressions of it. Thus, through her CEL Kate performs her social role in which she has invested herself (and which therefore matters to her) despite current challenges to it. Even though she consequently suppresses real feelings of anger, shame and anxiety, her 'self' is still authentic.

Kate's CEL represents her 'real' self, therefore. For example, in the beginning of the diary, when she suppresses feelings of shame, inadequacy and doubt, elicited as the result of bullying and induces feelings of anger and disgust at the bad behaviour of the other group of nurses, her CEL acts as a means of self-protection. It is one of the mechanisms by which she isolates herself from the bullies: protecting her 'self' from the imagined and actual judgements of others. At the same time, her CEL expresses her place in the hierarchy. Her CEL is an expression of self in which she recognises that she is seen as 'other'.

The CEL Kate carries out when she coaches the students in ECGs and handover reinforces her sense of identity as a professional nurse – restoring lost confidence and eliciting feelings of satisfaction and pride, emotions which she manages throughout her interaction with the students. Again, her CEL performs an aspect of her social identity as mentor that is regulated by her personal identity. Subsequently, in her growing realisation that she is ashamed about the other nurses, and in her deliberate inducement of anger and disgust at their behaviour, her CEL signifies an expression of shared identity in taking a share in her colleagues' 'immoral' behaviour. In this respect, Kate's CEL could be said to be an expression of other as self, in that as a nurse, she partakes in the shame of their unprofessional behaviour. Further, her CEL represents her professionalism in comparison to theirs, establishing and expressing a personal expression of identity within her social identity as a nurse.

It would appear that 'real' emotion is not always necessary to the expressions of identity (personal and social). The act of suppressing or inducing emotion in emotional labour can also be seen as expressing the 'real' self. Individuals have invested themselves in the social identities through which they perform their personal identity. This is where Hochschild's notion of emotion suppression, inducement and exhortation as a social under- standing of emotion is so important. Kate's CEL actually feeds and draws her into a closer awareness and experience of her emotion, and through that, her sense of self, in the emergence of her personal identity which animates the performance of her social identity. It would seem that the issues here are not to do with authenticity of emotion or self; they are to do with the acknowledgement and understanding of emotion and how we perceive them to reflect the self. This is about our ability to reflexively understand and manage our emotions as we interact and live our daily lives. It is this understanding that enables autonomy in our choices and actions.

The nature of collegial emotional labour in nursing

CEL demonstrates the link between personal identity and emotional labour, because the constraints of image and role, tied to social identity, are in the background; they do not dominate, as they do in TEL and IEL. The interplay and significance of emotions elicited from the natural, practical and social order are consequently more visible. Thus, to understand the relationship between emotions, emotional labour and identity, it is essential to first examine the interplay of emotions elicited in response to individual interactions and the overall context. *How* these emotions are reflected and refracted within the inner dialogue and then expressed or managed through acts of emotional labour subsequently becomes evident. Because the inner dialogue maintains a continuous and developing sense of personal identity, aspects of which are acted out through the individual's social identity, the relationship between emotion, emotional labour and identity is revealed.

Therapeutic, instrumental and collegial emotional labour all draw on deep and integral aspects of self (see Figure 9.1). However, Hochschild's notion of surface and deep acting, through which emotional labour is carried out, is inadequate to explain this process. The nature of the emotions elicited and managed, reflect different aspects of personal identity that are then expressed and performed using specific aspects of emotional labour that are related to social identity and role. These emotions might be suppressed or repressed, but this does not stop them from motivating action. If they are repressed or unacknowledged, they may also be difficult to manage or be unmanageable. These characteristics of emotion suggest that effective emotion management requires some reflexive acknowledgement of them. However, acknowledging emotions can be difficult. In Vignette 9, the diary provided a safe space in which Kate could express hers. This expression, however, does not bring immediate resolution; in a fragment of her inner dialogue, which takes place over ten days, she comes to see the importance of these emotions to her personal identity as it develops. Each individual story introduced and expressed, contributes to an overall story which mirrors a sense of self maintained and developed through her inner dialogue. Cognitive grappling, however, is not enough for Kate to come to terms with these painful issues; her outburst, in which they are expressed to relevant others, is also essential to this resolution.

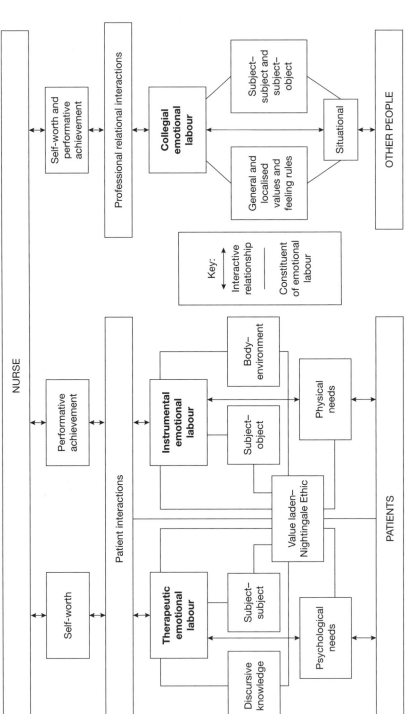

Figure 9.1 Typology of emotional labour

From this, several elements about emotional labour become clear. First, reflexive self-understanding and the expression of emotions suppressed for the purposes of role performance are essential. Emotions which are not inherently manageable and knowable coexist with, and must be managed alongside, those which are readily recognised, acknowledged and managed. Second, to be effective, emotional labour involves an ongoing process that is not specific to each individual act of emotional labour. Most importantly, negative emotions are not 'bad' emotions, or representative of an 'inauthentic' self. Rather, they can give an important insight into the self. Accepting these elements creates a position from which to challenge the circumstances in which emotional labour arises. Doing so, however, requires the acknowledgement that nurses are not perfect or equipped with the right emotion responses. Like their clinical skills, their emotional skills need to develop over time. By its very nature therefore, emotional labour in nursing challenges the professions image by questioning that nurses are born to nurse and are inherently good communicators. Their humanity is exposed for all to see, colleagues and patients alike. It is their humanity, predicated as it is in empathy, which ultimately enables them to offer emotional care.

Conclusion

CEL reveals that the management of emotions involves complex self-reflexive process, predicated within personal identity and expressed in social identity in microacts of emotional labour. Surface and deep acting as concepts are insufficient to explain this process. Chapter 10 puts together the different facets of emotional labour identified throughout the book and develops the notion of reflexive emotion management. The implications of this understanding of the nature of emotional labour in nursing are then considered.

Vignette 10 'The dying lady'

Kate: I was told [in handover] that somebody needed to get home because basically she is dying and she didn't want to go to the Hospice, she wanted to go home. So I made that my priority.

Catherine: So what did you do in order to deal with that?

Well, first of all I spoke to her and her husband and I said to them: 'Is this right, you want to get home? Do you want to get home a.s.a.p. or do you want to wait a week or two or three days, what do you want?' And he said, 'I want her home as soon as, tomorrow, Friday I want her home', and she said, 'Yes, let me go home'. So I then asked them if she had a Macmillan nurse, they said that she did. But they hadn't actually done much dealings with her for a long time and they couldn't remember her name. So they weren't really concentrating on what they wanted from the past, they were concentrating on each other for that moment. So I told them not to worry about it. So, I phoned the Hospice up and gave her name and her details and asked if I could get put through to the Macmillan nurses. They had a record of her, so I was then able to find out who her Macmillan nurse was. I then spoke to the doctor about getting her home the next day and we decided that we needed to get her home on good pain relief so that she was quite well controlled. Because even though she hadn't been taking pain relief, she was actually secretly in pain and wasn't telling anybody. So we spoke to her about that and I got the pain control nurse in so that we had her sorted out. Because of the fact that she had loose bowels it was decided that she would have Tylex because it has codeine in it and that might well tighten her bowels up a bit and also Amytriptoline to relax her at night to help her sleep. We thought we just need to get her through the weekend and give her everything for when their Macmillan calls on Monday. I gave them the name and the phone number of the Hospice obviously, so that if they had any problems they could sort that out over the weekend, because I didn't want them being left without any support. The pain control nurse came immediately, the doctor was there and didn't leave it [the TTOs], she was very good and got the TTOs [To Take Out: prescriptions for medication taken home] written up. So it was all established and I phoned up the Hospice again in reference for support for the weekend because I wanted to make sure that if anything happened then this couple would have support, because basically there is no Macmillan cover over the weekend but the Hospice has an on duty doctor who will go and call out if they have any problems. And I wanted to find out from my own point of view, 'cos

I've not done this before. So that was it really. I noted everything down. I put a note in the diary to get the lady a stretcher ambulance for that afternoon, and I informed the husband what I was doing and he went home and sorted their bedroom out so that they could get all the bed downstairs and move everything. It gave him enough time with her going home in the afternoon to get everything sorted out. I also talked to her about the pros and cons of taking the Tylex on a regular basis. 'Cos we deemed that she only had a maximum of about ten days, if she got a bit constipated then it really didn't matter it was just keeping her comfortable and the fact she had to take them. So I sort of gave her a good talk about analgesia and taking them on a regular basis and keeping the level up. From what I understand she went home yesterday. And that was my priority.

Why did you decide that this discharge procedure for this dying person was a priority over and above the other high dependency patients?

Because I think that care of the dying is as important as care of the living. Because I think that to die in a hospital bed when there's people quite willing to look after you at home is horrible. I think that too many people are allowed to die outside of their own home. I think too many old people are brought into hospital and are not allowed to die in peace at home as an old person. This lady wanted the comfort of her own home. If I were dying like that I'd want to be in my garden, in my bed, in my chair with people that I love. I wouldn't want to be in the humdrum of a busy acute surgical ward. I don't think that that is any place for anybody to die, not if you know they are dying and you can do something about it. And my other priorities, if anything else had happened and jumped in the way of that, then that would have changed. But as it happened I was able to make that my priority for most of the afternoon. I was also able to get people in there who also felt the same way. We all of us, the doctor, the pain nurse and her deputy and me, we all felt the same way: get this woman sorted out.

You mentioned that she was in secret pain. How did you know?

Basically because her family was telling us; some of the pain was hers and some was her family's. It doesn't matter, because when she was wincing they thought she was in pain and then they were in pain, because they can't control it. If they know she is being looked after and that she is being given the right pain control and they know the right rationale behind that, then they are more in power then, aren't they? You've given them something to help her. 'Cos I think that the worse thing for anybody who is a member of the family of somebody, who is dying, is not being able to do something, you know. And I believe in giving people power to be able to go and do something. Even if, for them, it is just to say to her, 'Are you in a little bit of pain?' And then ask the nurse: 'Can we get her something better for pain relief?' then I'll say: 'Yes, all right yes'. I'll give it a go; 'cos then they have done something haven't they? That is giving them all something, isn't it?

10 Reflexive emotion management

An attempt has been made to develop Hochschild's (1983) sociological concept of emotional labour through a theoretical and empirical exploration of its relationship with emotion and its application to nursing. The identification of therapeutic, instrumental and collegial aspects of emotional labour shows that Hochschild's concept can be developed and remains relevant to understanding the nature of emotional labour in nursing today. These three types of emotional labour have been developed by examining the relationship between emotion and emotional labour. This has involved a theoretical examination of the nature of emotion and how that might impact on the way emotion is elicited within interactive relationships. Recognising that emotion arises out of interaction and reflects and impacts on the nature of emotional labour has been a further means of developing the concept. These two approaches are interconnected as emotion is understood through biopsychosocial discourses, enabling holistic perspectives to be incorporated in the approach. Because the nature of emotion is relational and communicative, the interactional character of emotional labour has been developed. Developing a biopsychosocial and relational approach is essential to understanding emotional labour in nursing, because its practice and implementation within interactive relationships in nursing care is integral to it. Because emotion fundamentally informs personal identity, an exploration of the nature of emotion has enabled an evaluation of how emotional labour is integrally linked to personal identity and performed within socially prescribed nursing roles. This chapter puts these different components of emotion and emotional labour together and assesses how the concept has been developed by highlighting the main points drawn from the different theoretical approaches and underpinned and analysed through the empirical data represented in the vignettes.

Emotion

A central argument made throughout is that emotion management is about the management of *emotions*. Identifying what those emotions are is therefore absolutely crucial to understanding the process in which they are managed. However, care has been taken not to define emotion, because definitions are often limiting. In addition, the way in which emotions are expressed are often tangled up in feelings, thoughts and actions, described and made real through stories. In the empirical exploration of emotion, therefore, the emotion experiences of the nurses was examined. In order to identify emotion an attempt has been made to understand its nature as represented in theoretical discourses and examining them through the empirical data. Large extracts have been presented in the vignettes in order to represent those emotion stories in a way that the reader can engage with. A space within the text for the nurses' emotion experiences to emerge was created by the application of theory and reflexivity to the data which also provided a means to identify and analyse them.

The nature of emotion is multifaceted, theoretically represented across biopsychosocial discourses (S. Williams 2001). Emotion is primarily communicative, enabling individuals to situate and understand themselves in respect to the natural, material and social world around them, and with which they ceaselessly interact (Crossley 1998; Archer 2000). Emotions therefore arise through relational interaction. Because emotions are communicative and relational, they are linked to processes of cognition and therefore to conscious rational choice (Dewey 1922; Gerth and Mills 1964; Hochschild 1983; Denzin 1984; Scheff 1990; Csordas 1994; Greenwood 1994; Lazarus 1999; Eich et al. 2000; Gerrod Parrott 2001; Burkitt 2002). The relationship between emotion and language is central to the way in which individuals communicate (Eich et al. 2000). However, emotion can also be independent from cognition giving it the capacity to be revelatory without the need for cognitive understanding rooted in language (Freud 1915a, 1923; LeDoux 1998; Elster 1999, 2000; Turner and Stets 2005). Wentworth and Yardley argue that:

> Emotions are not inferential, as is symbolic language. Through emotion we may directly access the current physiological state of our bodies and minds, and are thus aware of the meaning of self-in-situation with quick, unfiltered immediacy. As presented to the self, emotion is the wisdom of the deeply social body derived from accumulated experience in the body social. The genius of our evolution is that bodily wisdom is not always 'appropriate', and by thus prying us out of a situated engulfment, inappropriate emotions may create a platform for individual perspective, reflexive self-consciousness, and creativity.
>
> (Wentworth and Yardley 1994: 37–38)

Because emotions are communicative, they are felt and experienced within the physical body and the psyche, understood and expressed through personal and social identity. Emotion is embodied through and within individuals. It is through emotion that individuals understand and gain knowledge of the ways of the world; emotion is what makes the relationship between them and the world 'real' (Denzin 1984; Stocker 1996). It is also through shared emotionality with others that individuals learn about their own and other's emotions. Transference is important to the process through which individuals learn about others in relation to themselves (Jacoby 1984; Stocker 1996; Craib 2001). Emotion allows individual salience to be recognised (Wentworth and Yardley 1994). Thus, linguistic and emotional experience, imagination and projection are integral to achieving individuation and establishing relationships with others. Without this ability, as is seen in those who have reduced emotion capabilities due to damage in their amygdala, extreme social impairment occurs, preventing the formation of social identity and interactive social relationships (Izard 1984; Wentworth and Yardley 1994; Stocker 1996; Goleman 1996, 1998; LeDoux 1998; Archer 2000; Turner and Stets 2005). Emotion is therefore crucial to identity and to social interaction.

> More specifically, human emotionality co-ordinates: the application of intelligence, long term memory, the salience of recognised individuals, intraindividual and intersubjective communication, social self-control through the agencies of empathy and conscience, the orientation of consciousness, and motivation.
>
> (Wentworth and Yardley 1994: 22)

Individuals however, cannot choose their emotions, but they do have *some* choice about how they respond to them (Elster 1999, 2000) and that choice is embedded within social relationships. Inducing emotion can also facilitate social interaction (Hochschild 1979, 1983). Thus, 'the interactive, relational character of embodied emotional experience and expression' facilitates autonomy in agency action. In this way 'embodied agency can be understood not merely as individual but also as institutional making' (Csordas 1994: 14; see also Lyon and Barbalet 1994): for the embodiment of emotionality emphasises 'the active, emotionally expressive body as the basis of self and sociality, meaning and order, set within the broader socio-cultural realms of everyday life' (Williams 1998c: 750–751).

Although emotion is communicative, it is not always understandable because it is not always linked to processes of cognition (Craib 1995, 2001). This is partly because emotion can be unconsciously experienced and partly because individuals are not always cognisant of their emotions (Craib 1995, 2001). It is also because emotion elicited within interactive relational situations, can respond to or change course as a result of the emotional state of others; this may occur directly, or through unconscious processes of projection and introjection (Bion 1979; Jacoby 1984; Spilius 1988; Joseph 1989; Klein, 1997; Craib 2001). Emotion therefore can be unmanageable and may be the impetus behind irrational acts or patterns of behaviour an individual might consciously wish they could overcome.

Thus, emotion is fundamentally communicative about self to self and self and other, whether that is people, things, nature or society. They are relational and interactive and emerge from relational interaction. The nature of emotion therefore is complex. To analyse the management of emotion without including an understanding of its nature would not only be reductive but to miss its significance.

Archer's (2000) notion of first and second order emotion offers a means by which individual emotions can be recognised and identified as they are elicited in relation to the interaction occurring and their import to the individual experiencing them. Emotion is elicited in response to different sources of interaction, which impact on whether it is manageable, and how and why it is managed. The value of identifying the source of the emotion can be seen in the analysis of Vignettes 7, 8 and 9. Identifying the source of emotion helped identify what emotions were present, and revealed different characteristics about the way in which they were managed. From this, different aspects of emotional labour and how they relate to nursing practice were identified. For example, TEL involves managing emotions elicited between nurse and patient or relative in the social order. IEL involves managing emotions elicited from the natural order in the patient and the practical order in the nurse. In CEL, the emotions arose from the social order. Identifying what the emotions are and whether they have been elicited from the natural, practical or social order is thus necessary to understanding the nature of the emotional labour being carried out.

However, first order emotion elicitation is still rooted in the social context within which the individual is interacting; and second order emotion which emerges as a result of the management process, and motivates social action, can only be understood from the context. Identifying and understanding that context as it pertains to the individual is also essential to situating that experience and understanding subsequent emotion expression. Feeling rules encapsulate the socio-cultural relevance of the context to emotion experience and expression. For example, in Vignette 10, 'The dying lady', the emotions identified are from the social order. But the significance of the emotions is understood through the social context and with those she is interacting with; conceptualised in the notion of feeling rules. As a result, Kate's emotion management in her interaction with the dying lady is indicative of TEL and with her colleagues, as CEL.

Feeling rules

Feeling rules have two essential characteristics (Hochschild 1983). The first is that they represent the currency of feeling owed in transactions between people. The second is that they help define and identify the feelings and emotions being experienced through the context in which they are taking place. Within these characteristics, feeling rules represent the interactional and relational nature of emotion as something that is shared and meaningful beyond that of the individual. The natural, material and social world, with which the individual interacts, is to a degree external to them. Feeling rules are therefore an inherently social manifestation of emotion. Seeing feeling rules as extrinsic to individuals and wholly intrinsic to social values, norms and ideology however, both reifies them and detracts from their crucial interactional and relational characteristics. Feeling rules are understood, learnt, passed on and acted upon through outward interaction within relationships between individuals. Individuals therefore do not interact with feeling rules; they interact with other individuals who like them, have internalised these rules within their explicit and implicit, cognitive and emotion memory (Giddens 1979, 1992). Hochschild (1983) represents this understanding in her notion of deep acting, where the individual has worked on their emotions so much that they actually believe the emotions they are expressing. Similarly, Archer (2000) notes that individuals need to have invested themselves in those activities and beliefs to which feeling rules are relevant for that internalisation to matter to them. Feeling rules, therefore, do not define emotions or feelings. They represent something that is infinitesimally social and external to the individual yet something intrinsically personal, internalised by the individual. However, the sociological significance of feeling rules only becomes relevant when interaction occurs. Thus, feeling rules represent aspects of social structure, which Williams, drawing on Giddens' notion of structuration, notes 'may fruitfully be seen as both the *medium* and the *outcome* of the emotionally embodied practices it recursively organises' (S. Williams 1998b: 125, original emphasis).

Feeling rules represent the currency of feeling which individuals feel they owe or are owed by another in their social exchanges. In Vignette 7, Emily believed that she owed it to her patient to explain why walking out to the bathroom was an important part of post-operative recovery. Her TEL involved her suppressing feelings of annoyance that this patient was being intransigent in order to secure her cooperation with this aspect of her care. It was an expression of Emily's internalised belief in the feeling rule that nurses' TEL involves educating patients in order to facilitate their health and wellbeing. The patient, on the other hand, cared less about this particular feeling rule despite cooperating in the first instance. It was the feeling rule that represented the belief that nurses offer a safe space in which patients can express their feelings and worries (also pertinent to TEL) that mattered to her. The currency in the feeling exchange between the two was affected by what each brought to the dynamic interaction. Their emotions were not defined by the feeling rules; rather, they informed the individual of aspects of those feeling rules which were important to them. Through their emotions, 'the meaning of self-in-situation' in which emotions and feeling rules bring meaning, was directly accessed (Wentworth and Yardley 1994) and brought to the dynamic between them.

Because feeling rules are a way in which individuals understand what the currency of feelings owed in interaction are, they are related to issues concerning power and status (Wouters 1991). In therapeutic and instrumental emotional labour, power is located within the image and social role of nurses and within the structures and organisation of the institutions within which health care is practised. Thus, feeling rules associated with them are both general and specific because they are applicable to all involved while also relating to particular aspects of the nurse's role. Status and power reside within the roles of nurse and patient. The nurse has power as a result of her knowledge and skill, and status in her professional role of nurse. The patient or relative has less because of their very need for that knowledge and skill. Because there is an uneven distribution of power in the relationship, the profession of nursing has a responsibility to uphold the quality and degree of knowledge and skill of its practitioners, and hold their care to account. This is why in the UK nurses undergo three-year training programmes before becoming registered practitioners. Once on the NMC Register they become accountable for their practice in accordance with the NMC Professional Code of Conduct. Individual nurses then have a responsibility to maintain their registration. Thus within the profession, the practice of nursing care is taught and monitored. Emotional labour as a component of that care is included within these structures. This is most evident in IEL, which is taught as a component of clinical skills. The patients for whom Kate passed an NG tube in Vignette 8, for example, trusted in her clinical skills and her emotional labour expertise. They were vulnerable and reliant on her ability to do so. Kate held power over them. However, the onus was on her to ensure that her skill and knowledge was good enough to practise on her patients. Kate understood this, describing it as the art and science of nursing. The feeling rules relevant to IEL reflect this power balance; the patient trusts the nurse to carry out invasive procedures on their physical body in a way that minimises their discomfort through their practical skill and their empathy for their predicament. The nurse believes that this is essential to being able to efficiently carry out such procedures and understands the ordeal it must be for the patient. The feeling rules represent the emotion exchange between nurse and patient. Part of that exchange includes the currency of feeling owed; the nurse owes expert care, skill and empathy and the patient owes trust and gratitude.

The feeling rules represent issues relating to power and status, but actual power is exercised in the interaction that takes place between individuals and within groups. This was seen in Vignette 7, where Emily's patient made her vulnerable to her by exercising her right to complain about the care given. This was a very effective use of emotion to challenge the power Emily held while asserting her status as an individual patient. Emily's own physical emotion response illustrates this. However, the traditional balance of power between nurse and patient was eventually re-established as a result of the two individual personalities involved and the relationship they forged through their interaction. This example demonstrates where feeling rules are both external and internalised. The external nature of feeling rules helps shape the boundaries within which interaction takes place enabling shared understanding. However, each individual brings their own interpretation of those feeling rules, representing their personal investment in them. Individuals' autonomy of action, and their ability to affect change, is exercised through their action and interaction, mediated by external and internalised feeling rules, norms and values.

How power and autonomy are linked to individual personal identity and exercised in social interaction is more visible in CEL. For example, in Vignette 9, Kate's collegial emotional labour initially represented her acceptance of the status given to her by the other nurses, but over a period of time she challenged it. Through that process she asserted her own personality and understanding of her social role as a nurse. This process was an internal one; her CEL being predicated on internalised feeling rules representing status and place, reproduced consistently in her interactions with her colleagues. Feeling rules therefore, are implicated in personal and social identity. This is evident in Vignette 10. Here Kate has internalised the feeling rules about nurses managing their emotions to facilitate a peaceful and dignified death for their patients. In her interaction with her colleagues, Kate can act on this internalised feeling rule by asserting the priority of this patient's care needs because the feeling rule is also external, representing shared boundaries in which Kate and her colleagues work together. Thus, the doctor and pain control nurse work with Kate, their CEL bound by common values. In doing so, they exercise their power to change the care offered to the dying woman and her family, but they do so in a way that acknowledges and respects their individual needs and human dignity.

Personal identity and the inner dialogue

Hochschild (1983) believes that emotional labour draws on an individual's deep and integral sense of self. Because feeling rules that shape emotional labour are prescribed, monitored and controlled for commercial purposes, emotional labour becomes exploitative, resulting in an inauthenticity of emotion expression and self-alienation. Evidence of the exploitative nature of emotional labour is clearly visible in nursing too. However, changes in social expectations of nursing care need to be balanced with the need and vulnerability of those who require it. Hochschild identifies that commercial companies exploit emotional labour by teaching and monitoring it. Indeed, Smith (1992) also identifies the importance of teaching emotional labour to nurses, not as a means of exploiting them, but as a means of enabling their abilities. However, it is difficult for this not to result in their exploitation when the nurse draws on a sense of self that is personal and integral to them but that they have to fit into feeling rules which dictate what they should be feeling. As has been suggested throughout, a possible resolution to this difficulty can be found in understanding more fully the relationship between personal identity and emotional labour.

Archer (2000) suggests that an individual's personal identity is shaped and continuously developed and reflected on through their inner dialogue. The inner dialogue also comments on and works towards maintaining a balance between first order emotions elicited as a result of interaction with the social, material and natural world. Second order emotion arises from this reflexive inner dialogic process. The emergence of second order emotion represents the process through which individuals manage their emotions. This management is directly linked to personal identity; aspects of which are acted out through their social roles and identities to which emotional labour is connected. Emotional labour therefore, not only draws on an individual's sense of self: it is dependent on it. Thus, emotional labour stems from the individual's continuous and constantly developing personal identity, of which a conscious awareness is created through their internal conversation.

Establishing a therapeutic relationship between nurse and patient depends upon fostering maturity and forward personality development in the nurse (Peplau 1988). Thus, not only is there a direct connection between identity and emotional labour, but also the degree of self-awareness of the individual carrying it out is central to its process and success. In Vignette 10, Kate needs a degree of self-awareness to recognise and understand the needs of the dying woman and her family. In fact, she demonstrates a remarkable degree of empathy and self-awareness in her account of how her actions and care impacts on them. This is particularly evident in her detection of the family's pain and loss of power in controlling the dying woman's pain. This stems from her personal identity for the kind of care given is an extension of herself; another nurse may not be able to accomplish this level of empathy, as is the case with Susan in Vignette 4. In order to facilitate such emotional labour, therefore, the emotional capacity of the individual is crucial.

The inner dialogue

Archer's (2000) notion of the inner dialogue offers a means of analysing the conceptualisation of the self and how emotional labour draws on it. Two important ideas need to be considered in respect to this. The first is that the nature of emotion impacts on its management. The second is that the individual needs to have invested themselves in the situations and relationships in which they are interacting. Both of these are linked to past experiences which have helped forge their personal identity. Archer's use of Peirce's inner conversation between the 'I', 'me' and 'you' representing different stages of the ego's dialogue dovetails with Hochschild's notion of a prior self which impacts on the present self's interpretation of current events. However, it is Archer's inner dialogic process of discernment, deliberation and dedication, predicated on cognitive processes, that reveals the means by which second order emotion is reached.

Cognitive appraisal can take place instantly, representing well-trodden pre-reflexive patterns of behaviour and understanding laid down in the implicit and explicit memory. Archer links this primarily to emotions elicited in the practical order which are largely pre-reflexive in nature. However, pre-reflexive, habitual patterns of behaviour can relate to the social order too. Thus, in Vignette 9, Kate's CEL represented a well-practised response to her low place in the hierarchy (a response indicating the internalisation of feeling rules). Likewise in Vignette 7, Emily did not exercise a great deal of thought in her TEL when explaining why it was necessary that her patient walked out to the toilet. This may have contributed to her failure to detect her patient's distress.

The inner dialogue can also comment on pre-reflexive actions while they are being carried out. As well as being immediately relevant, this commentary can also contribute towards a wider overarching one, continuous and developing over a significant period of time. Thus, in Vignette 9, at the same time as carrying out each pre-reflexive act of CEL, Kate's inner dialogue commented on those behaviour patterns, and the emotions they elicited in her, in respect to each microact. These in turn contributed towards a larger commentary that put together each microact in an overall understanding of her personal identity. This longer process ultimately resulted in her challenging her low place in the hierarchy and facilitated the reassertion of her personal identity, expressed through her newly established social identity as an alpha senior nurse. Different expressions of CEL, which represented her new place, resulted from this.

The dialogic process here represents the nature of emotion across the passage of time. Emotions can be elicited, experienced and acted upon instantly. They can also be the impetus to actions over a short period of time, or ongoing emotions sustained over an extended period of time. Understanding the nature of emotion is also necessary to understanding this process in other ways. Intense emotion sustained over a lengthy period of time appeared to cause Kate to become ill. In this case, emotion could be said to embody the social as she embodied her social situation within these sustained emotions (Lyon and Barbalet 1994; Lupton 1998). Emotions elicited in response to the natural order can bypass cognitive process altogether, causing immediate visceral response. However, visceral response is not limited to emotion elicited from the natural order. Kate lost control of her emotions during handover, when they erupted from her, causing visible distress and further embarrassment.

Emotions elicited from the practical order can balance out subjective emotions elicited from the social order. This is particularly evident in the discernment, deliberation and dedication phases of the inner dialogue seen in Vignettes 8 and 9. In Vignette 8, the success that Kate experienced in passing the NG tube gave perspective on the doctor's probable response when the second patient pulled it out. Likewise in Vignette 9, the satisfaction Kate derived from mentoring the students and in caring for the woman with a CVA helped her balance the import of her shame and anger experienced as a result of bullying. These emotions are significant because they are not dependent on subjective interpretation; they are understood as being true because they are elicited in response to objects which cannot have a subjective opinion. Thus, these emotions act as an objective commentary on the inner dialogue as it considers what matters to it, how much it cares and what the cost of its choices will be. However, they can contribute to this process *only if they are acknowledged.*

One of the fundamental difficulties with Archer's notion of the inner dialogue is that it requires the individual to have a conscious recognition of their emotions. The whole dialogic process can fall down at the discernment phase. Irrespective of whether they are elicited from the natural, practical and social order, acknowledgement of emotions is essential to the inner dialogue. This is where Hochschild's notion of emotion exhortation and Freud's understanding of conscious ideational presentation of repressed emotions become important to the process. For example, in Vignette 5 Maxine deliberately exhorts her feelings of satisfaction in successfully caring for her patients, as does Kate towards the end of Vignette 9. This exhortation of emotion is necessary to Maxine's identity because it enables her to find a degree of perspective in her response to the bullying she has experienced. In conjunction with her emotion imagination in which she projects her feelings on to those who have hurt her, Maxine is able to reach the dedication phase in which she realises that giving into the bullying will result in the loss of her satisfaction and pride in nursing. Thus, second order feelings of pride emerge outweighing her feelings of uncertainty, and she is able to dismiss the other nurses' actions and opinions. As Hochschild (1983) notes, emotion exhortation can be achieved by drawing on past experiences, but it can also specifically help in the management of emotions that support the self as it is understood in relation to others. Thus, emotion exhortation is directly linked to the establishment and maintenance of personal identity.

Projection and introjection of emotion are also important to the inner dialogic process. In Vignette 9, in order to re-establish a positive sense of self, Kate adopted an 'I-It' attitude in her relationship with the students. She did this by projecting her own learning needs on to them, and introjecting theirs in turn. In doing so, she objectified them in response to her own unconscious need to counter the criticisms of the other nurses (Buber 1922; Jacoby 1984; Craib 2001). Emily also adopted the 'I-It' attitude with the patient who made a complaint about her in Vignette 7. Her purpose was always to vindicate herself and protect her no-complaints record. She did not adopt an 'I-Thou' attitude and relate to the genuine otherness of her patient. However, as Jacoby (1984) notes, this does not prevent the 'I-It' relationship from having a mutual benefit, as seen when the patient felt that her concerns were eventually listened to.

In Vignette 5, Maxine developed an 'I-Thou' relationship with the nurses who attempted to bully her. This did not mean that she empathised with them, but that she allowed herself to connect with their genuine otherness. This meant she opened herself up to acknowledging their rejection of her.

In order to do this she needed to own her personal feelings, needs and values in order to reject the judgements of the others. Maxine drew on fantasy and past emotion experiences to achieve this. In her imagination she acted out a scenario where she reversed their act of bullying making them recognise their need of her. Thus, Maxine was able to consider the viewpoint of the others without losing herself to it in the process. In the deliberation and dedication phase of the inner dialogue she is able to assess how much the actions of the other nurses matter to her and what the cost of her response will be. She realises that her sense of self is strong enough to sustain their act of aggression, without this damaging her personal identity. Thus, the process of emotion projection and imagination provides a sense of 'self-in-situation' that facilitates cognitive understanding – and is therefore necessary to the dialogic process.

However, in Vignette 4 when Susan attempted to use her emotion imagination to achieve the 'I-Thou' attitude and empathise with her patient's sister, she was unsuccessful because she was unable to acknowledge her real feelings of anger towards her. Instead, the ideational presentation of herself as a kind, responsible nurse – an internalised feeling rule – resulted in her conscious mind interpreting her anger as guilt and repressing her anger. As a consequence, during the interview several months after the event, Susan was still unconsciously expressing anger and interpreting it as guilt. This is indicative of a feedback loop within the inner dialogue. Here, the conscious discernment, deliberation and dedication phase goes round and round in a loop, unable to reach second order emotion because of its inability to recognise the actual source of the dominating emotion. Thus, Susan felt a continuing sense of guilt about her lack of care for both the patient and her sister despite her reasoning telling her this was not the case. The feedback loop can be broken, as Kate demonstrates in Vignette 9. However, in this case, this took place over a substantial period of time and the spontaneous outburst of emotion expression represented a crucial turning point. The expression of the emotion appeared to result in a conscious acknowledgement of it (Lupton 1998), enabling Kate to break the shame spiral.

Adopting an 'I-It' or 'I-Thou' attitude is a part of self-reflexivity (Jacoby 1984; Prus 1996). In order to develop 'I-It' or 'I-Thou' relationships, processes of projection and introjection, components of transference, are necessary (Jacoby 1984; Craib 2001). Thus, it seems that transference is part of the discernment, deliberation and dedication phase of the inner dialogue. Within the vignettes, transference is connected to emotion memory, imagination and the ability to exhort or induce emotion. The internalisation of feeling rules is a part of this, as they also represent a sense of emotion owed to others. This can elicit within the self the need to exhort emotion or draw on emotion memory or imagination. This is clear in Vignette 10, in Kate's empathy with the dying woman and her family. She imagines how she would feel dying on a busy surgical ward. To understand a sense of emotion owed to others, without that requiring a negation of the self, a successful confluence within the inner dialogue is required: when this occurs individuation is achieved.

> Individuation is a matter of my understanding my own uniqueness and individuality through my relationships with and dependence upon others. It involves recognising that there are essential ways in which I am dependent on all other people, that I share a common humanity with others and that I can only know myself through recognising and finding my place within *and* against them.
>
> (Craib 2001: 187, original emphasis)

In Vignettes 5 and 9 respectively, Maxine and Kate's emotional reflexivity represents a successful confluence of emotion within their inner dialogues, and the achievement of individuation. With Kate, this took place over a passage of time; with Maxine, it was expressed in a moment in the diary but following events that took place eight hours earlier. Processes of transference within their inner dialogue were identified in both, and appear to be necessary to the accomplishment of the inner dialogic process. Individuation involves an acknowledgement of personal identity set against one's place in the social world; that acknowledgement is acted out through different sets of social identities, such as mother, daughter, nurse and partner. As mother or daughter, emotion work stems from that personal identity, as nurse, emotional labour does. Where individuation was not achieved, as in the case of Susan in Vignette 4 and Emily in Vignette 7, this appeared to be due to a lack of confluence within the inner dialogue. In Susan's case this was because she was unable to acknowledge her anger and became trapped in a feedback loop, unable to recognise the genuine otherness of the patient's sister without that impacting negatively upon her own sense of self. Ultimately she adopted an 'I-It' attitude, separating herself from her own emotions and using them to motivate her to learn from the situation. In Emily's case, she used the 'I-It' attitude to achieve her goal of maintaining her no-complaints record, drawing on her excellent communication skills to do so. She was so successful that the patient rescinded the complaint, believing that her concerns had been considered. However, Emily did not relate to her genuine otherness and was unable to understand herself in respect to her patient or recognise her role in the patient's initial distress. This was evident in her inner dialogue by the absence of her 'you' projecting into the future. In Vignette 10, individuation is seen in Kate's ability to recognise her empathy, and her need to help the dying woman without introjecting her patient's need into herself and losing her sense of personal identity. She recognises her common humanity with them, while acknowledging her place in respect to theirs.

Reflexive emotion management

An exploration of the nature of emotion in respect to the inner dialogue has revealed how individuals draw upon their personal identity in their acts of emotional labour. Hochschild (1983) suggests that individuals manage emotional labour through surface and deep acting. She suggests that in surface acting individuals suppress their real emotion and express another in its place, deceiving others about their real feelings. In deep acting, by working on their emotions, individuals successfully deceive themselves and believe the emotions they express are genuine. They know what emotions to express through feeling rules. This is because for Hochschild, feeling rules in emotional labour dictate which emotions should be expressed in each individual's surface and deep acting.

Emotional labour is shaped by social role, and therefore the social identities each nurse has as a nurse. This is where feeling rules in their external function shape the boundaries of social interaction. However, emotional labour itself involves interaction. Personal identity emerges during interaction between individuals in which emotional labour is carried out. Each person, nurse, patient, relative, colleague brings their unique self to that interaction. Personal identity animates surface and deep acting either by expressing or defending its sense of self. Equally surface and deep acting may express the degree to which individuals wish to share their self with those they are interacting with: it is expressive of the private/public distinction.

Surface acting and personal identity

In surface acting this distinction can result in the expression of an entirely professional persona in which the nurse successfully hides her real emotions. This could be because she is defending her sense of self due to the unreasonable expectations or attitudes of others – as Amelia does in Vignette 2. Whereas Emily in Vignette 7 uses surface acting when she is pleasant and polite when confronting the patient about her complaint, her real feelings are expressive of her personal identity and animate her surface acting. The patient knows that Emily is upset about her complaint; it is motivating her to confront her! Susan's personal identity also animates her surface acting in her interaction with her patient's sister, who both accuses her of being a murderer and later apologises for it. She is polite and accepting on the surface, but neither person is deceived about their real emotions.

Surface acting may also animate and defend the self at the same time. This is the case in Kate's CEL when she suppresses her feelings of misery, but also uses her CEL to demonstrate her acceptance of the place the other nurses have given her. In fact, if she was not able to do this, their bullying would be unsuccessful; the other nurses would not be able to see the results of their actions and the use of emotion as status markers (Clark 1990) would not be possible. Thus, while Kate acts in such a way as to accept her exclusion, her shame and hurt are also visible. Surface acting in which real feelings are hidden may also be an expression of personal identity which has internalised the belief that a professional nurse does not show her real feelings – as Paris does in Vignette 1. Here Paris chooses to keep her private self separate from her relationship with her patients, whereas another nurse might share or let her personal distress show in order to demonstrate her empathy with her patient's emotional needs that she is unable to fulfil.

The suppression of surface emotions does not necessarily represent inauthentic emotion expression. Rather, in Vignette 2, Amelia uses her surface acting to defend her self from Alix's dad's aggression; her real emotions inform her about the degree of threat she feels. In Emily's case her real emotions motivate her choice of action in confronting the patient and defending her no-complaints record. In Vignette 4, if Susan's real emotions had not animated her surface acting, it would have made a mockery of the awfulness of what had occurred for both her and the patient's sister. In Kate's situation they both express her place and status, and protect her from further denigration. In Vignette 1, if Paris had not managed her feelings of distress, she would be aggrieved at her lack of professionalism: her surface acting therefore is expressive of her belief that the expression of her feelings is not helpful to the patient. This is where deep acting can also take place at the same time as surface acting. The act of suppressing surface emotions does not prevent the nurse from drawing on other, more deeply felt emotions which motivate her care, and express her sense of self.

Deep acting and personal identity

Deep acting is deeply expressive of the self. This is particularly evident in Vignette 10, when Kate engages and commits herself fully to the needs of the dying woman and her family. Her TEL involves her relating to the genuine otherness of her patient's impending death and how this might make her family feel. Kate's empathy is profound, based on personal experience and deeply expressive of her personal identity. She is immediately concerned about facilitating the family's wants, in providing background support, immediately available when needed. She empathises with their pain, their need for privacy, their need for control. Her approach to the patient's pain needs includes that of the family's pain. She facilitates a frank conversation to alleviate their concerns about the drugs' side effects. Her deep acting is indicative of projection when she identifies the family's need to be in control to be able to do something for their dying member. She recognises their need to be alone, to make the most of the time they have together, the need to die at home surrounded by familiar comforts. She draws on their need to have support available for when they do not know what to do. She works with the husband in organising the stretcher ambulance so that he has time to make arrangements at home. At the same time she wants to learn about how to facilitate such care – another central aspect of her personality seen in

Vignettes 8 and 9. Kate brings her whole self to her care of this patient. She is not deceiving or pretending in any way. Her personal identity infuses and animates her deep acting in her role as nurse working towards facilitating a peaceful and dignified death for her patient – an internalised feeling rule pertinent to TEL. She reflexively manages her emotion*s*. She uses her own personal experience to motivate her care and empathise with their situation. She carries out TEL and CEL in her interactions with them and her colleagues.

Authenticity of self in emotional labour

Authenticity of self in emotional labour is not necessarily connected to the suppression or repression of emotion; nor does the expression of negative emotions necessarily lead to self-alienation. Authenticity of self in emotion is about the capacity of the individual to identify, acknowledge and understand their emotions. It is about their ability to reflexively manage them; it is about their understanding of the emotions of others; and it is about having a maturity of self that realises the impact they have on others and others have on them. This understanding of self conceptualised here as personal identity, is what the individual draws on when they carry out emotional labour, shaped by their social identity as a nurse.

When nurses express their increasing frustration and dissatisfaction at the level of emotional care they give due to lack of time, or fear of abuse or complaint, they are not expressing alienation from their sense of self; they are directly identifying which aspects of nursing they no longer find satisfying. These are authentic and legitimate feelings. When Paris cries with distress at not being able to give good psychological care to her patients in Vignette 1, her emotions express to her how important that aspect of her identity is. When Amelia withholds her empathy from Alix's dad in Vignette 2, even though she knows his need, it is because her emotions inform her about how uncomfortable he makes her feel; they tell her she cannot trust him and that this frustrates her because she knows it affects the quality of care he receives. When Susan cries to her mum after an awful shift in which she has been accused of being a murderer in Vignette 4, it expresses her confusion and hurt. These emotion experiences represent authentic legitimate emotions that demonstrate how much nurses care. Although these are negative emotions and although they suppress their real feelings in their acts of emotional labour, it does not result in inauthenticity and self-alienation. Rather, those feelings and actions inform and motivate them to realise their discomfort of the social situation or their relationships with those they care for or work with. It is the relationships and social situations that they perceive as being inauthentic. Thus, they feel they cannot represent their personal identity in such situations – eliciting negative, yet nonetheless real, emotions. That many nurses feel they are being inauthentic to themselves due to expressing surface emotions they do not really feel, is indicative of their

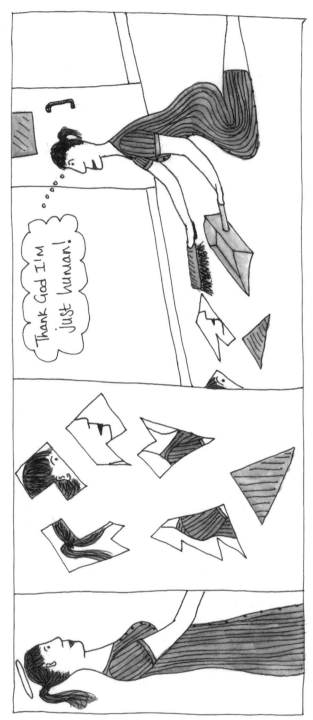

'The perfect nurse'

increasing need to defend themselves from the onslaught of public abuse. That they recognise their discomfort in doing so, suggests that their sense of self is intact.

The nature of emotional labour in nursing: implications for practice

In therapeutic emotional labour, the balance of power between the nurse and patient or relative and the status of the nurse has been upset in some instances. This affects the currency of feeling owed for both parties. The introduction of quasi-market principles and patient 'rights' has changed the nature of the exchange between nurse and patient. It has shifted the balance of power towards the patient. Rather than creating a more equal partnership, the exercise of the patient's right to complain questions the nurse's knowledge and skill, which in turn challenges their status as a trustworthy professional. In Vignette 2, Amelia exclaims: 'they wouldn't believe us, they don't believe you'. This breaks the feeling rule in which the patient believes they can trust the nurse – and the nurse acts to uphold that trust. This is not just because there is now a system in place through which patients can make complaints. However, the system does support a changing attitude within society in which the practice of health care has been made more accountable to the public. Increased accountability is necessary. However, patients are not the same as consumers. They are vulnerable individuals, the majority of whom have no choice but to accept the available care on offer. They are caught in a position in which they have little control and have to trust. As Giddens (1992: 138) notes, 'to trust the other is also to gamble on the capability of the individual to actually be able to act with integrity'. Trusting the nursing care on offer should not be a gamble. Registered nurses have a responsibility to provide optimum care and to act with integrity towards their patients. To suggest that nurses do not do so would be a gross exaggeration. However, the evidence suggests that feeling rules pertinent to therapeutic emotional labour have been challenged by nurses as well as by patients.

Feeling rules relating to therapeutic emotional labour include teaching about health care, listening to patient concerns and supporting dying patients. Teaching about health care is perceived as a central tenet of health promotion – an important component of nursing care. Supporting the dying is also something that nurses consider essential. However, listening to their patients' concerns is sometimes given less priority. Paris identifies this in Vignette 1. In Vignette 2 no effort was made by any of the nurses (not just Amelia) to find a way in which Alix's dad could express his anger. In Vignette 7, Emily did not in the first instance use the opportunity to walk the patient to the bathroom to find out about her real anxieties, nor does she evidence any empathy when the patient manipulates her into doing so. While nurses frequently do carry out TEL, it is also being undercut by changing priorities, attitudes and values.

There are three essential ways in which nursing can work towards addressing this problem. First, acknowledgment that nursing care is a collaborative partnership, in which nurse and patient work together to develop a therapeutic relationship, is needed. This awareness needs to be actively incorporated into the profession's wider relationship with society as well as in actual nursing care. It is not just a case of making it clear that abuse towards nurses will not be tolerated – although this is important too; it is in helping people realise that care in the twenty-first century is as much about the person receiving it as the person giving it. As Peplau notes:

> the nursing process is educative and therapeutic when nurse and patient can come to know and to respect each other, as persons who are alike, and yet different, as persons who share in the solution of problems.
>
> (Peplau 1988: 9)

When Rowan Williams (2006) makes a passionate plea to nurses to remember the human dignity of their patients, it is important that those who seek care remember that nurses are people too; respect is necessary for patient and nurse alike.

Second, TEL needs to be actively reintegrated into general nursing care, taught and monitored in the same way that IEL is. This will entail accepting the increased pace of nursing work and throughput of patients, and the development of nursing care towards more clinical and managerial roles. TEL has traditionally been seen as a part of hands-on nursing care; since nurses are still involved in this part of practice, TEL should continue to be incorporated here. However, there is no reason why this should be the only place within the nursing process that TEL is relevant. Where appropriate all other components of nursing care can include opportunities for TEL. However, it needs to be accepted that these will not provide extended sessions for patients due to time limitations; rather than bewailing this, nurses need to work together in providing their patients with a safe space to confide their anxieties and worries. They also need to look at how this can become a shared responsibility with allied health care professionals. Effective communication and good CEL are essential to this process. Further research is required into the most effective ways TEL can be reintegrated into nursing care.

Third, understanding that emotional labour not only is integrally linked to, but also flows from personal identity, is important in how the profession teaches and monitors it. Emotional labour does not involve a simple suppression of one's own emotions in order to facilitate the right emotional response in others. It requires complex emotional reflexivity where the nurse's real emotions need to be acknowledged rather than denied – even though in the act of emotional labour they may suppress them. As professionals, nurses have a responsibility to use their emotional skills in situations where those they care for are vulnerable and in need. Being able to understand one's own

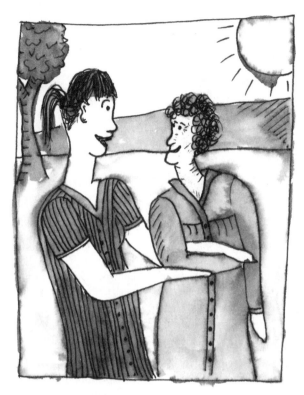

'Working together'

emotions and how they affect one is important in helping others to identify theirs and considering how they might manage them. This is what makes emotional labour in nursing so crucial. It is because that understanding is there, that IEL is so effective. Introducing and teaching emotional labour skills to student nurses is essential, but so too is fostering the development and maturity of nurses into reflective practitioners able to 'apply principles of human relations to the problems that arise at all levels of experience' (Peplau 1988: xi). As Hochschild so wisely notes, this takes work.

Bibliography

Adams, A., Bond, S. and Hale, C. (1998) 'Nursing organisational practice and its relationship with other features of ward organisation and job satisfaction', *Journal of Advanced Nursing*, 20: 1212–1222.

Archer, M. (2000) *Being Human: The problem of agency*, Cambridge: Cambridge University Press.

Barbalet, J. M. (2001) *Emotion, Social Theory and Social Structure*, Cambridge: Cambridge University Press.

Barbalet, J. (ed.) (2002) *Emotions and Sociology*, Oxford: Blackwell.

Bendelow, G. and Williams, S. (eds) (1998) *Emotions in Social Life*, London: Routledge.

Bion, W. R. (1979) 'Making the best of a bad job', unpublished lecture to the British Psycho-Analytical Society, cited in N. Symington (1986) *The Analytic Experience: Lectures from the Tavistock*, London: Free Association Books.

Bolton, S. (2000) 'Who cares? Offering emotion work as a "gift" in the nursing labour process', *Journal of Advanced Nursing*, 32(3): 580–586.

Bolton, S. (2001) 'Changing faces: nurses as emotional jugglers', *Sociology of Health and Illness*, 23(1): 85–100.

Bolton, S. and Boyd, C. (2003) 'Trolley dolly or skilled emotion manager? Moving on from Hochschild's Managed Heart', *Work, Employment and Society*, 17(2): 289–308.

Bone, D. (2002) 'Dilemmas of emotion work in nursing under market-driven health care', *International Journal of Public Sector Management*, 15(2): 140–150.

Bourdieu, P. (1990) *The Logic of Practice*, Oxford: Polity.

Bowers, K. S. (1984) 'On being unconsciously influenced and informed', in K. S. Bowers and D. Meichenbaum (eds) *The Unconscious Reconsidered*, New York: Wiley.

Buber, M. (1922) *I and Thou*, translated by W. Kauffmann (1991), New York: Free Press.

Burkitt, I. (1997) 'Social relationships and emotions', *Sociology*, 31(1): 37–55.

Burkitt, I. (2002) 'Complex emotions: relations, feelings and images in emotional experience', in J. Barbalet (ed.) *Emotions and Sociology*, Oxford: Blackwell.

Cacioppo, J. T. and Petty, R. E. (1981) 'Lateral asymmetry in the expression of cognition and emotion', *Journal of Experimental Psychology: Human Perception and Performance*, 7: 333–341.

Clark, C. (1990) 'Emotions and micropolitics on everyday life: some patterns and paradoxes of "place"', in T. Kemper (ed.) *Research Agendas in the Sociology of Emotions*, Albany, NY: State University of New York Press.

Cooley, C. H. (1902) *Human Nature and the Social Order*, revised edition 1922, New York: Charles Scribner's Sons.

Cornelius, R. (1996) *The Science of Emotion: Research and tradition in the psychology of emotions*, Upper Saddle River, NJ: Prentice Hall.

Craib, I. (1994) *The Importance of Disappointment*, London: Routledge.

Craib, I. (1995) 'Some comments on the sociology of emotions', *Sociology*, 29(1): 151–158.

Craib, I. (1998) 'Sigmund Freud', in R. Stones (ed.) *Key Sociological Thinkers*, Basingstoke: Palgrave.

Craib, I. (2001) *Psychoanalysis: A critical introduction*, Cambridge: Polity.

Crossley, N. (1998) 'Emotion and communicative action', in G. Bendelow and S. Williams (eds) *Emotions in Social Life*, London: Routledge.

Csordas, T. (1994) *Embodiment and Experience: The existential ground of culture and self*, Cambridge: Cambridge University Press.

Darwin, C. (1955 [1872]) *The Expression of the Emotions in Man and Animals*, New York: Philosophical Library.

Davies, C. (1995) *Gender and the Professional Predicament in Nursing*, Buckingham: Open University Press.

de Laine, M. (2000) *Fieldwork, Participation and Practice*, London: Sage.

Denzin, N. (1984) *On Understanding Emotion*, San Francisco, CA: Jossey-Bass.

Department of Health (DoH) (1995) *The Patient's Charter and You*, London: DoH.

Department of Health (2000) *The NHS Plan: A plan for investment a plan for reform*, London: HMSO.

de Raeve, L. (2002) 'The modification of emotional responses: a problem for trust in nurse–patient relationships?', *Nurse Ethics*, 9: 465–471.

de Swaan, A. (1990) *The Management of Normality: Critical essays in health and welfare*, London: Routledge.

Dewey, J. (1922) *Human Nature and Conduct: An introduction to social psychology*, New York: Holt.

Duck, S. (1998) *Human Relationships*, London: Sage.

Eich, E., Kihlstrom, J., Bower, G., Forgas, J. and Niedenthal, P. (2000) *Cognition and Emotion*, Oxford: Oxford University Press.

Elster, J. (1999) *Alchemies of the Mind: Rationality and the emotions*, Cambridge: Cambridge University Press.

Elster, J. (2000) *Strong Feelings*, Cambridge, MA: MIT Press.

Fineman, S. (ed.) (1993) *Emotion in Organisations*, London: Sage.

Folkman, S. and Lazarus, R. (1988) 'The relationship between coping and emotion: implications for theory and research', *Social Science and Medicine*, 26(3): 309–317.

Foucault, M. (1978) *The History of Sexuality. Volume 1: An introduction*, London: Penguin.

Fox, N. (1993) *Postmodernism, Sociology and Health*, Buckingham: Open University Press.

Fox, N. (1995) 'Post modern perspectives on care: the vigil and the gift', *Critical Social Policy*, 15(44): 107–125.

Freud, S. (1915a) 'The unconscious', in J. Strachey (ed.) *Standard Edition*, Vol. 14: 159–217, London: Hogarth Press, cited in A. Hochschild (1983) *The Managed Heart*, Berkeley, CA: University of California Press.

Freud, S. (1915b) 'Instincts and their vicissitudes', *Standard Edition*, Vol. 14: 109–140.

Freud, S. (2001 [1923]) *The Ego and the Id*, London: Vintage.

Freud, S. (1925) *An Autobiographical Study*, *Standard Edition*, Vol. 20: 1–74.

Freund, P. (1990) 'The expressive body: a common ground for the sociology of emotions and health and illness', *Sociology of Health and Illness*, 12(4): 452–477.

Gerrod Parrott, W. (ed.) (2001) *Emotions in Social Psychology*, Philadelphia, PA: Taylor & Francis.

Gerth, H. and Mills, C. W. (1964) *Character and Social Structure: The psychology of social institutions*, New York: Harcourt, Brace and World.

Gerth, H. and Mills, C. W. (1991) *From Max Weber: Essays in sociology*, London: Routledge.

Giddens, A. (1979) *Central Problems in Social Theory: Action, structure and contradiction in social analysis*, London: Macmillan.

Giddens, A. (1990) *The Consequences of Modernity*, Cambridge: Polity.

Giddens, A. (1992) *The Transformation of Intimacy: Sexuality, love and eroticism in modern societies*, Cambridge: Polity.

Goffman, E. (1956) 'Embarrassment and social organisation', *American Journal of Sociology*, 62: 264–271.

Goffman, E. (1959) *The Presentation of Self in Everyday Life*, New York: Doubleday Anchor.

Goffman, E. (1961) *Encounters*, Indianapolis, IN: Bobbs-Merrill.

Goffman, E. (1967) *Interaction Ritual*, New York: Doubleday Anchor.

Goffman, E. (1969) *Strategic Interaction*, Philadelphia, PA: University of Pennsylvania Press.

Goffman, E. (1974) *Frame Analysis*, New York: Harper Colophon.

Goleman, D. (1996) *Emotional Intelligence: Why it can matter more than IQ*, London: Bloomsbury.

Goleman, D. (1998) *Working with Emotional Intelligence*, London: Bloomsbury.

Graham, H. (1983) 'Caring: a labour of love', in J. Finch and D. Groves (eds) *A Labour of Love: Women, work and caring*, London: Routledge & Kegan Paul.

Greenwood, J. (1994) *Realism, Identity and Emotion*, London: Sage.

Henerson, M. E., Morris, L. L. and Fitz-Gibbon, C. T. (1987) *How to Measure Attitudes*, Newbury Park, CA: Sage.

Hetherington, K. (1998) *Expressions of Identity: Space, performance, politics*, London: Sage.

Hochschild, A. (1975) 'The sociology of feeling and emotion: selected possibilities', in M. Millman and R. Kanter (eds) *Another Voice*, Garden City, NY: Anchor.

Hochschild, A. (1979) 'Emotion work, feeling rules and social structure', *American Journal of Sociology*, 85: 551–575.

Hochschild, A. (1983) *The Managed Heart*, Berkeley, CA: University of California Press.

Hochschild, A. (1990) 'Ideology and emotion management: a perspective path for future research', in T. Kemper (ed.) *Research Agendas in the Sociology of Emotions*, Albany, NY: State University of New York Press.

Hopfl, H. and Linstead, S. (1993) 'Passion and performance: suffering and carrying of organisational roles', in S. Fineman (ed.) *Emotion in Organisations*, London: Sage.

Huxley, E. (1975) *Florence Nightingale*, London: Chancellor Press.

Izard, C. E. (1984) 'Emotion-cognition relationships and human development', in C. E. Izard, J. Kagnan and R. Zajonc (eds) *Emotions, Cognition and Behaviour*, New York: Cambridge University Press.

Jacoby, M. (1984) *The Analytic Encounter: Transference and human relationship*, Toronto: Inner City Books.

James, N. (1989) 'Emotional labour: skill and work in the social regulation of feelings', *Sociological Review*, 37: 15–42.

James, N. (1992) 'Care = organisation + physical labour + emotional labour', *Sociology of Health and Illness*, 14(4): 488–509.

James, V. and Gabe, J. (1996) *Health and the Sociology of Emotions*, Oxford: Blackwell.

James, W. (1884) 'What is an emotion?', *Mind*, 9: 188–205.

Joseph, B. (1989) 'Transference: the total situation', in M. Feldman and E. B. Spilius (eds) *Psychic Equilibrium and Psychic Change: Selected papers of Betty Joseph*, London: Routledge.

Katz, J. (1999) *How Emotions Work*, Chicago, IL: University of Chicago Press.

Kemper, T. (1978) 'How many emotions are there? Wedding the social and the autonomic components', *American Journal of Sociology*, 93(2): 263–289.

Kemper, T. (ed.) (1990) *Research Agendas in the Sociology of Emotions*, Albany, NY: State University of New York Press.

Kihlstrom, J., Mulvaney, S., Tobias, B. and Tobias, I. (eds) (2000) 'The emotional unconscious', in E. Eich, J. Kihlstrom, G. Bower, F. Forgas and P. Niedenthal, *Cognition and Emotion*, Oxford: Oxford University Press.

Kikumura, A. (1998) 'Family life histories: a collaborative venture', in R. Perks and A. Thomson (eds) *The Oral History Reader*, London: Routledge.

Klein, M. (1997 [1955]) 'On identification', in M. Klein, *Envy and Gratitude and Other Works 1946–1963*, London: Vintage.

Layder, D. (2004a) *Emotion in Social Life*, London: Sage.

Layder, D. (2004b) *Social and Personal Identity*, London: Sage.

Lazarus, R. (1982) 'Thoughts on the relationship between emotion and cognition', *American Psychologist*, 37: 1019–1024.

Lazarus, R. (1991) *Emotion and Adaptation*, London: Oxford University Press.

Lazarus, R. (1999) *Stress and Emotion: A new synthesis*, London: Free Association Books.

LeDoux, J. (1996) *The Emotional Brain: The mysterious underpinnings of emotional life*, New York: Simon & Schuster.

LeDoux, J. (1998) *The Emotional Brain*, New York: Phoenix.

Lewis, H. B. (1971) *Shame and Guilt in Neurosis*, New York: International Universities Press.

Lupton, D. (1996) 'Your life in their hands: trust in the medical encounter', in V. James and J. Gabe (eds) *Health and the Sociology of Emotion*, Oxford: Blackwell.

Lupton, D. (1998) *The Emotional Self*, London: Sage.

Lyon, M. and Barbalet, J. (1994) 'Society's body: emotion and the "somatization" of social theory', in T. Csordas (ed.) *Embodiment and Experience*, Cambridge: Cambridge University Press.

McClure, R. and Murphy, C. (2007) 'Contesting the dominance of emotional labour in professional nursing', *Journal of Health Organisation and Management*, 21(20): 101–120.

MacKay, L. (1989) *Nursing a Problem*, Milton Keynes: Open University Press.

MacKay, L. (1993) *Conflicts in Care: Medicine and nursing*, London: Chapman and Hall.

MacKay, L. (1996) 'Nursing and doctoring: where's the difference?', in K. Soothill, C. Henry and K. Kendrick (eds) *Themes and Perspectives in Nursing*, London: Chapman and Hall.

McNeese-Smith, D. (1999) 'A content analysis of staff nurse descriptions of job satisfaction and dissatisfaction', *Journal of Advanced Nursing*, 29(6): 1332–1341.

Maggs, C. J. (1980) 'Nurse recruitment to four provincial hospitals in 1881–1921', in C. Davies (ed.) *Rewriting Nursing History*, London: Croom Helm.

Majomi, P., Brown, B. and Crawford, P. (2003) 'Sacrificing the personal to the professional: community mental health nurses', *Journal of Advanced Nursing*, 42(5): 527–538.

Mead, G. H. (1934) *Mind, Self and Society*, edited by C. W. Morris, Chicago, IL: University of Chicago Press.

Mills, C. W. (2002 [1951]) *White Collar: The American middle classes*, Oxford: Oxford University Press.

Minister, K. (1991) 'Feminist frame for the oral history interview', in S. B. Gluck and D. Patai (eds) *Women's Words*, London: Routledge.

Montgomery, A., Panagopolou, E., de Wildt, M. and Meenks, E. (2006) 'Work–family interference, emotional labour and burnout', *Journal of Managerial Psychology*, 21(1): 36–51.

Morrison, M. and Galloway, S. (1996) 'Researching moving targets: using diaries to explore supply teachers' lives', in E. S. Lyon and J. Busfield (eds) *Methodological Imaginations*, London: Macmillan.

Nightingale, F. (1980 [1859]) *Notes on Nursing: What it is and what it is not*, Edinburgh: Churchill Livingstone.

Olesen, V. and Bone, D. (1998) 'Emotions in rationalizing organizations: conceptual notes from professional nursing in the USA', in G. Bendelow and S. Williams (eds) *Emotions in Social Life*, London: Routledge.

Peirce, C. S. (1998) *Collected Papers of Charles Sanders Peirce*, Volume 4, *The Simplest Mathematics*, edited by C. Hartshorne, P. Weiss and A. W. Burkes, Bristol, UK: Thoemmes Continuum.

Peplau, H. (1988 [1952]) *Interpersonal Relations in Nursing*, Basingstoke: Palgrave Macmillan.

Philips, S. (1996) 'Labouring the emotions: Expanding the remit of nursing work', *Journal of Advanced Nursing*, 24: 139–143.

Plummer, K. (2001) *Documents of Life 2*, London: Sage.

Prus, R. (1996) *Symbolic Interaction and Ethnographic Research*, Albany, NY: State University of New York Press.

Reader's Digest (1993) *Complete Word Finder*, edited by S. Tulloch, London: Reader's Digest Association.

Salvage, J. (1985) *The Politics of Nursing*, Oxford: Butterworth Heinemann.

Sandelands, L. and Boudens, C. (2000) 'Feeling at work', in S. Fineman (ed.) *Emotion in Organisations*, London: Sage.

Schacter, D. (1987) 'Implicit memory: history and current status', *Journal of Experimental Psychology: Learning, Memory and Cognition*, 13: 501–518.

Scheff, T. (1990) 'Socialization of emotions: pride and shame as causal agents', in T. Kemper (ed.) *Research Agendas in the Sociology of Emotions*, Albany, NY: State University of New York Press.

Schwartz, G. E., Davidson, R. J. and Maer, F. (1975) 'Right hemisphere lateralization for emotion in the human brain: interaction with cognition', *Science*, 190: 286–288.

Smith, P. (1991) 'The nursing process: raising the profile of emotional care in nurse training', *Journal of Advanced Nursing*, 16: 74–81.

Smith, P. (1992) *The Emotional Labour of Nursing*, London: Macmillan.

Spilius, E. B. (ed.) (1988) *Melanie Klein Today: Developments in theory and practice*, Vol. 2, London: Routledge.

Stocker, M. (1996) *Valuing Emotions*, Cambridge: Cambridge University Press.

Strongman, K. T. (1987) *The Psychology of Emotion*, 3rd edn, Chichester: Wiley.

Strongman, K. T. (2003) *The Psychology of Emotion*, 5th edn, Chichester: Wiley.

Symington, N. (1986) *The Analytic Experience: Lectures from the Tavistock*, London: Free Association Books.

Taylor, C. (1985) *Human Agency and Language*, Cambridge: Cambridge University Press.

Theodosius, C. (1998) 'The developing remit of nursing during the last thirty years', unpublished paper, Essex University.

Theodosius, C. (2006) 'Recovering emotion from its management', *Sociology*, 40(5): 893–910.

Tonkin, E. (1992) *Narrating our Past*, Cambridge: Cambridge University Press.

Turner, J. (2000) *On the Origins of Human Emotions: A sociological enquiry into the evolution of human affect*, Stanford, CA: Stanford University Press.

Turner, J. and Stets, J. (2005) *The Sociology of Emotions*, Cambridge: Cambridge University Press.

Walby, S. and Greenwell, J., with MacKay, L. and Soothill, K. (1994) *Medicine and Nursing: Professions in a changing health service*, London: Sage.

Wentworth, W. and Yardley, D. (1994) 'Deep sociality: a bioevolutionary perspective on the sociology of human emotions', in D. Franks, W. Wentworth and J. Ryan (eds) *Social Perspective on Emotion*, Greenwich, CT: JAI Press.

Williams, R. (2006) 'Personal is professional', *Church Times*, 19 May.

Williams, S. (1998a) 'Arlie Russell Hochschild', in R. Stones (ed.) *Key Sociological Thinkers*, Basingstoke: Palgrave.

Williams, S. (1998b) '"Capitalising" on emotions? Re-thinking the inequalities in health debate', *Sociology*, 32(1): 121–139.

Williams, S. (1998c) 'Modernity and the emotions: corporeal reflections on the (ir)rational', *Sociology*, 32(4): 747–769.

Williams, S. (2001) *Emotion and Social Theory*, London: Sage.

Witz, A. (1992) *Professions and Patriarchy*, London: Routledge.

Wouters, C. (1989a) 'The sociology of emotions and flight attendants', *Theory, Culture and Society*, 6: 95–123.

Wouters, C. (1989b) 'Response to Hochschild's reply', *Theory, Culture and Society*, 6: 447–450.

Wouters, C. (1991) 'On status competition and emotion management', *Journal of Social History*, 24(4): 669–717.

Zajonc, R. B. (1984) 'On the primacy of affect', *American Psychologist*, 39(2): 117–123.

Index

Note: Page numbers in bold refer to figures or tables.

Adams, A. 171
'Alix's Dad' vignette 27–8; advancement
    and speed-up of nursing 46; authentic
    emotions 215; feeling rules 35–6; image
    and identity 32–3, 106; ongoing,
    relational interaction 113; private-public
    realm 40; surface acting 40, 213, 214;
    trust and power in emotional labour
    42–3, 217
allocation of work 129–31, 132
anticipation 72, 78, 93
Archer, Margaret 59, 61, 79, 122, 124,
    125, 141, 148, 152, 164, 188, 193,
    202, 203, 204, 205, 208; differences in
    approach to Hochschild 90, 91–2, 96–7,
    100, 105–12; model of emotion 90–114
articulation-rearticulation process **100**,
    101, **109**, 110, 111, 183
audio diaries 122–4
authenticity: and CEL 178, 193–5;
    deception 79; emotional 47; of self in
    emotional labour 215–17; repression
    and suppression of emotion 108; self
    awareness/reflexivity 195
autonomy 98, 207; in CEL 193–5; in IEL
    170–1; in TEL 152–4
'Average shift' vignette 117–19, 121, 123

Barbalet, J.M. 183, 184, 189, 203, 209
Being Human 90
Bendelow, G. 62
biological approach to emotion 56–61, 62,
    69, 87
biomedical model 59, 161
Bion, W.R. 139, 203
biopsychosocial approach to emotion 52,
    73, 86, 90, 201, 202
bodies 33–4
body-environment 91, **93**, 105, 162, **163**
Bolton, S. 34, 37, 39, 42, 47
Bone, D. 32, 37, 39, 45, 46, 106, 168
Boudens, C. 133, 135, 136, 183

boundaries, narrative 135; in 'The Breaking
    the Shame Spiral' vignette 183–5; in
    'The Complaint' vignette 148–9; in
    'The NG Tube' vignette 162–4
Bourdieu, P. 79
Bowers, K.S. 57
Boyd, C. 42
'Breaking the shame spiral' vignette 174–7;
    authenticity and autonomy of self
    193–5; bullying 183, 184, 190, 194,
    209, 213; CEL 181, 182–92, 195, 209,
    213; identifying the source of emotion
    204; inner dialogue 209–10, 211, 212
Buber, Martin 137, 210
bullying 126, 128, 129, 130, 132–3;
    'Breaking the shame spiral' vignette 174,
    176, 183, 184, 190, 194, 209, 213; *see
    also* 'Maxine's rant' vignette
Burkitt, I. 105, 180, 202

Cacioppo, J.T. 58
'Care of the dying' vignette 198–200; deep
    acting and personal identity 214–15;
    emotion management 204; empathy 214;
    inner dialogue 208, 211, 212;
    internalised feeling rules 207, 211;
    self-awareness 208
caring 33–4, 171, 172
Clark, C. 132, 184, 185, 213
clinical nursing skills 113, 161, 170, 173;
    IEL an integral component 161–2, **163**,
    165, 168; status 44, 166
cognition and emotion 49–64, 202; and
    biological approach 56–61, 62, 69, 87;
    Hochschild's linguistic argument 52–6,
    62
cognitive appraisal 53, 55, 57–8, 61, 62–3,
    69, 93, 99, 208–9
cognitivism 91
collegial emotional labour (CEL) 178–97,
    182; authenticity and autonomy of self
    193–5; in 'Breaking the shame spiral'

vignette 181, 182–92, 195, 209, 213;
comparisons with TEL and IEL 180–1;
feeling rules 180, 181, **182**; first order
emotion 190–1; inner dialogue 183,
184–5, 190–2, 195, 209–13; in nursing
195–7; personal identity and 178, 182,
183, 184, 207; power and autonomy
207; and reintegrating TEL into nursing
care 218; social identity and 182, 183,
184; social order emotions 182, 188,
204
communication skills 143, 144, 162, 163,
170, 173, **182**
'Complaint, The' vignette 142; feeling rules
205; identifying the source of emotion
204; inner dialogue 209, 210, 212;
power and status 206; surface acting
213; TEL in 147–51, 154–5, 209, 217
conformity 70–1, 83
conscious awareness 80, 91, 93, 94, 101,
140, 208
consumer-oriented approach in the NHS
37, 43
Cooley, C.H. 139
Cornelius, R. 53
counsellors 145, 169
Craib, I. 75, 139, 140, 150, 203, 210, 211,
212
Crossley, N. 202
Csordas, T. 202, 203

Darwin, Charles 51, 68–9, 73, 75
data, analysing 133–41; narratives 133–6;
reflexivity 136–9, 140; theoretical
frameworks 140–1; transference 139–40
data collection: *see* research methods
Davies, C. 33, 41, 44, 169, 172
de Laine, M. 123
de Raeve, Louise 154, 155
dedication phase 101, 102, 104, 151, 191,
209, 210, 211
deep acting 18–20, 77, 78–80, 86, 100,
105; and emotion memory 78, 79, 81–3,
105, 108; of flight attendants 23;
inauthenticity and self-deception 23, 75,
79, 85; links to method acting and
dramaturgy 73–4; and personal identity
213, 214–15
deliberation phase 101–2, 103–4, 191, 208,
209, 211
Denzin, N. 152, 202, 203
Department of Health (DoH) 37, 44, 173
Dewey, J. 51, 70, 202
diaries, audio 122–4
discernment phase 101, 102–3, 191, 208,
210, 211
discursive order: *see* social order
division of labour 44, 45

Duck, S. 77
dying, care of the 217; *see also* 'Care of the
dying' vignette
dynamic tensions in narratives 135; CEL in
'The Breaking the Shame Spiral' vignette
185–9; IEL in 'The NG Tube' vignette
164–5; TEL in 'The Complaint' vignette
149–50

education role in nursing 145–6
ego 69, 71, 74, 85, 100, 101, 105, 140
Eich, E. 202
elicitation-expression 70, 87
Elster, J. 202, 203
emotion: Archer's model of 90–114;
expression of 41–2; gendered
characteristics 24–5; and language 202;
nature of 91, 201–4; trajectories across
time 92, 98, 110, 124, 209; *see also* first
order emotion; second order emotion
emotion elicitation 90, 91, 93, 100, 105,
108, 114
emotion exchange 34–6, 40, 43, 63, 206;
and emotional labour 48, 113–14
emotion exhortation 108, 114, 194, 210
emotion management 6, 14–16, 21, 61, 75,
84, 110, 112–13, 204; in the absence of
emotional labour 5–6; anger 183–4; in
Freud's analysis 84, 85; private 19, 22;
reflexive 201–19; and
repressed/suppressed emotion 84, 195;
and self-reflection 156; separation from
emotional elicitation 90, 105; *see also*
fear management
emotion memory 80–3, 93, 109–10, 111;
deep acting and 78, 79, 81–3, 105, 108;
explicit 80, 81, 85, **109**, 209; implicit
80, 85, 108, **109**, 209
emotion orders 93
emotion work 15, 32, 69, 71, 72, 73,
104, 193; as a commodity 37; in the
private-public realm 15, 36–40;
transmutation to emotional labour 20,
39, 40, 193; as women's work 24, 212;
in the workplace 19, 20
emotional communiqués 133, 183
emotional labour 5–6, 20–1; authenticity of
self in 215–17; as a commodity 15, 22,
37, 39, 43, 47; devaluing of 5, 44, 45;
differences between flight attendants and
nurses 33, 35, 42, 48, 52, 53, 62, 113;
and emotion exchange 48, 113–14; and
gender 24–6; Hochschild on 13–26,
29–30, 39, 42, 201; linked to hands-on
nursing care 44–5, 171, 218; in nursing
29–30, 34–5, 47–8, 106, 217–19;
and personal identity 218–19; in the
private-public realm 15, 36–40;

problems of marginalisation 5–6, 47–8, 156, 168–9, 172, 217–19; requires time 45, 46, 170; significance of 26; teaching to nursing students 30, 32, 41, 155; transmutation from emotion work to 20, 39, 40, 193; trust and power 40–3, 48, 113, 127; typology of **196**; *see also* flight attendants' emotional labour
'emotional micropolitics' 132
empathy 138, 208
essentialism 91
ethical consent 7
explicit memory 80, 81, 85, **109**, 209
Expression of the Emotions in Man and Animals, The 68

fear management 55–6, 59, 60–1, 93, 162
Feedback Theory 58
feeling rules 16–18, 26, 33–6, 75, 204–7; to alleviate shame and embarrassment 41; and building relationships on trust 41, 48; in CEL 180, 181, **182**; challenges to 37, 39, 217; in IEL 162, **163**, 167; internalisation 78, 79, 81–3, 205, 207; optional 96–7; in personal and social identity 207; related to issues of power and status 205–7; in TEL **147**, 217
Fineman, S. 29, 120
first order emotion 90, 92–9, 141, 190–1, 204; and emotion memory 108; and inner dialogue **100**, 101, **109**; and the vomiting patient 105–6
flight attendants' emotional labour 20, 22–3, 25, 31; differing from that of nurses 33, 35, 42, 48, 52, **53**, 62, 113; inauthenticity 39; surface acting 77
flight or fight response 58, 60, 87, 93
Folkman, S. 53
Foucault, Michel 41
Fox, N. 34
Freud, Sigmund 51, 100, 184, 202; synthesising with interactionism 69, 75, 78, 83–4, 87, 108–9; transference 140; and the unconscious 83–6, 87, 106, 108, 114, 210
Freund, S. 62, 79

Gabe, J. 62
Galloway, S. 122, 123
gender 24–6, 212
Gerrod Parrott, W. 202
Gerth, H. 51, 70, 161, 202
gestures communicating emotion 68–9
Giddens, A. 41, 205, 217
goal-oriented action 161
Goffman, Erving 15, 18, 51, 70–1, 73, 77, 83, 97
Goleman, D. 203

Graham, Hilary 172
Greenwell, J. 167, 171, 181
Greenwood, J. 202
growth (movement) in narratives 135; CEL in 'The Breaking the Shame Spiral' vignette 189–90; IEL in 'The NG Tube' vignette 165–8; TEL in 'The Complaint' vignette 150–1

'Half measures' vignette 11–12, 113, 124, 215, 217; advancement and speed-up of nursing 46; emotion management 16, 21; emotional labour 21, 106; emotional labour and gender 25–6; feeling rules 17–18; inauthenticity of self 24; surface and deep acting 19–20, 214
handovers 3–4, 16, 174, 175–6, 177, 179, 189, 194
hands-on nursing care 44–5, 46, 129, 171, 172, 218
Henerson, M.E. 123
Hetherington, K. 193
Hochschild, Arlie Russell 39, 42, 68, 69, 70, 78, 81, 83, 141, 153, 155, 193, 194, 195, 202, 203, 204, 205, 210, 213; background 13–14; developing a sociological understanding of emotion 51–2; differences in approach to Archer 90, 91–2, 96–7, 100, 105–12; emotional labour 13–26, 29–30, 39, 42, 201; engaging with the biological approach to emotion 56–7, 59, 62, 69; linguistic argument of emotion 52–6, 61–2; new social theory of emotion 51, 62–4, 68, 71–6, 86–7; synthesising Darwin and Freud with interactionist theory 68–87
holistic care 43–4, 48, 87, 143, 144
Hopfl, H. 132
Huxley, E. 31

'I-It ' 137, 140–1, 153, 187, 188, 210, 211, 212
'I-Thou' 138, 140–1, 154, 187, 210–11
'I', 'you' and 'me' 100, 101, 208
id 69, 71, 74, 83–4, 85, 100, 101
id-ego-superego 85, 87, 114
Ideology and emotion management 77
implicit memory 80, 85, 108, **109**, 209
inauthenticity: and exploitation in emotional labour 208; Hochschild's emotional labour 22, 24, 39, 193; nurse's emotional labour 45; self deception in 'The murderer' vignette 76; women's emotional labour 25
individuation 61, 203, 212
inner dialogue 91, **100**, 101–4, 106–7, 141, 208–12; in audio diaries 122; in CEL 183, 184–5, 190–2, 195; difficulties with

109, 210; in IEL 167; links to personal identity 100, 207–8; negative feedback **109**, 110, 114, 211; passage of time 109–10; second order emotion 100–1

instrumental emotional labour (IEL) 161–73, **196**; autonomy and investment of self in 170–1; comparisons with CEL 180–1; differences between TEL and 172–3; emotions in 162, 204; feeling rules 162, **163**, 167; 'NG tube' vignette 162–70, 171; in nurse-patient relationship 161–2, 164; in nursing 171–4; and personal identity 162, 164, 170–1, 172; power and status 206; source of emotions 204

interactionist theory: and Hochschild's new social theory of emotion 71–80; synthesising with the organismic school 70–1; synthesizing Freud with 69, 75, 78, 83–4, 87, 108–9

interpersonal communication skills 143, 144, 162, **163**, 170, 173, **182**; in TEL **147**

interviews 124–5, 133

introjective identification 140, 187, 210–11

Izard, C.E. 58, 93, 203

Jacoby, M. 137, 138, 139, 140, 153, 203, 210, 211

James, Nicky 45, 46, 171

James, V. 62

James, William 58, 69, 169

Joseph, B. 140, 203

Katz, J. 152–3, 183, 184

Kemper, T. 183, 188

Kihlstrom, J. 80

Kikumura, A. 125

Klein, M. 140, 203

Layder, D. 77

Lazarus, R. 53, 56, 57, 202

LeDoux, J. 57, 58, 60, 80, 81, 85, 93, 202, 203

Lewis, H.B. 148, 183, 184

linguistic argument of emotion 52–6, 61–2

Linstead, S. 132

'Looking Glass Self' 139

Lupton, D. 33–4, 40, 62, 149, 189, 209

Lyon, M. 203, 209

MacKay, L. 44, 167, 168, 181

Macmillan nurses 11, 20, 41, 198

Maggs, C. 31, 37

Majomi, P. 45

Managed Heart, The 14, 59, 77; Appendix A 51, 56–7, 61, 64

'Maxine's rant' vignette 88–9, 130, 132; achieving invidiation in 212; emotional

exhortation 210; first order emotion 98–9; 'I-Thou' attitude 210–11; inner dialogue 102–4, 122, 210–11, 212; integrating Hochschild and Archer in analyzing 110–12

McClure, R. 47

McNeese-Smith, D. 171

Mead, G.H. 51, 70, 83, 84, 100

mentoring students 123–4, 174–6, 187–8

Mills, C.W. 14, 51, 70, 161, 202

Minister, K. 125

Montgomery, A. 45

moral responsibility 154–6

Morrison, M. 122, 123

'Murderer' vignette 65–7; authentic emotions 214, 215; deep acting and emotion memory 81–3; Freud and the unconscious 86; 'I-It attitude' 212; 'I-Thou' attitude 211; inauthenticity and self-deception 76; inner dialogue in 211, 212; moral responsibility 155–6; new social theory of emotion in 72–3, 76; surface acting 78, 214

Murphy, C. 47

narratives 133–6; analysing 'The Breaking the Shame Spiral' vignette 182–92; analysing 'The Complaint' vignette 147–51; analysing 'The NG Tube' vignette 162–9

National Health Service: commercialisation of health care 5; consumer-oriented approach 37, 43; increased workload and shorter in-patient stays 44, 45; NHS Plan 37, 44

natural order 92–3, **93**, 98, 105–6, 113, 162, 204, 209

negative emotions 56, 197, 215

neuroscience 58, 59, 60, 62, 80, 85

'NG tube' vignette 158–60, 204, 206, 209; IEL in 162–70, 171

NHS Plan 37, 44

'Nightingale Ethic' 31, 37, 41, 147, 153, 156, 169, 192

Nightingale, Florence 31, 145, 168, 169

nurse-doctor relationship 168, 179–80, 181

nurse-patient relationship: emotion exchange 34–6, 40, 43, 63, 206; essential role of emotional labour 34–5; in IEL 161–2, 164; impact of nurse's personality/behaviour 155, 164; self-awareness 146, 207, 208; status and power 37, 39, 40, 42–3, 182, 206, 217; therapeutic 33, 37, 47, 48, 63, 146–7, 154, 206, 218; trust in the 40, 41, 43, 48, 113, 217

nurses: abuse towards 5, 32, 43, 215, 217, 218; changing role of 44, 45; emotional

labour differing from that of flight attendants 33, 35, 42, 48, 52, 53, 62, 113; image and identity 30–3; juggling work 45; motivation for becoming 171; pay 36–7; personality 155, 156; stress and burnout 45
nursing: addressing the problems of TEL 5–6, 47–8, 217–19; art and science of 168, 169; emotional labour in 29–30, 47–8, 106, 217–19; hands-on care 44–5, 46, 129, 171, 172, 218; moral responsibility 154–6; nature of CEL in 195–7; nature of IEL in 171–4; nature of TEL in 154–7, 172; role of education 145–6; speed-up and advancement 24, 43–6; status 26; surgical 161; *see also* clinical nursing skills
Nursing and Midwifery Council (NMC) Code of Conduct 30, 206

Olesen, V. 45, 106
organismic school 51, 57, 58, 62, 70–1, 86

patient choice 37, 42
patient complaints 42, 43, 149–50, 217
patients: demanding emotional labour as a commodity 37, 39; emotions in hospital 5; teaching independence to 145–6; vulnerability 5, 41, 42, 48, 63, 113, 217
Patients' Charter 37, 44
Peirce, Charles 100–1, 107, 208
Peplau, Hildegau 143, 145, 146, 155, 156, 164, 170, 208, 218, 219
performative concerns 93–4
personal identity 30–3, 92, 94, 97, 153, 162, 164; and authenticity of the self 193, 194; and deep acting 213, 214–15; emergence from second order emotion 105, 106, 148; emotional labour flowing from 218–19; and feeling rules 207; links to CEL 178, 182, 183, 184, 207; links to IEL 162, 164, 170–1, 172; links to inner dialogue 100, 207–8; and reflexive emotion management 213; and surface acting 213–14
personality 155, 156
Petty, R.E. 58
Philips, S. 44, 45, 169, 172
physiological experience 62, 69, 72, 74
Plummer, K. 122
Portman, Alice 143
possibility in narratives 135–6; CEL in 'The Breaking the Shame Spiral' vignette 190–2; IEL in 'The NG Tube' vignette 168–9; TEL in 'The Complaint' vignette 151
power: in CEL 207; in emotion exchanges 34, 35; in IEL 206; in the nurse-patient

relationship 37, 39, 40, 42–3, 182, 206, 217; related to feeling rules 205–7; and social status 42; in TEL 206, 217; and trust in emotional labour 40–3, 48, 113, 217
practical order 93, 93–5, 98, 113, 162, 164, 188, 189, 209
pre-reflexive behaviour 79, 80, 82, 94, 164, 168, 208–9
preceptors 121
private/public emotion 97
private/public realm 15, 36–40, 97
Project 2000 44
projective identification 140, 210–11
Prus, R. 125, 136, 137–8, 139, 211
psychoanalysis 57
psychological care 11–12, 17, 21, 26, 43, 46, 144, 215; in the 'Nightingale ethic' 156; and well-being 145, 146, 147, 165, 172
psychology 57, 84
psychotherapy 140, 145, 169
public emotion 97, 193

racial prejudice 111
reflexive emotion management 201–19
reflexivity 99, 100, 109, 136–9, 140, 148–9, 218
repressed emotion 83, 84, 106–7, 108, 183–4, 195, 210
research methods 6–7, 120–5, 135; audio diaries 122–4; interviews 124–5, 133; participant observation 120–2; researcher's relationship with the nurses 121, 122, 124, 125, 137–8
researcher-nurse, role of 136–7

Salvage, J. 169
Sandelands, L. 133, 135, 136, 183
Scheff, T. 148, 183, 184, 202
Schwartz, G.E. 58
'Scrotal drain' vignette 49–50; biological approach to emotion and cognition 60–1; linguistic argument of emotion 55–6; problems with Hochschild's theory of emotion in analyzing 62–3; representation of natural order in 98
second order emotion 90, 99–101, 108, 148, 184, 192, 204; emergence of personal identity 105, 106, 148; and the inner dialogue 100–1, 109; time trajectories 98
self: authenticity and autonomy in CEL 193–5; authenticity in emotional labour 215–17; inauthenticity of 22–4, 25, 39, 40, 45, 47, 76, 193, 215; investment in IEL 170–1; investment in TEL 152–4; notion of the 75; real and false 84, 85, 87, 100, 193

self-alienation 208, 215
self-awareness 146, 207, 208
self-deception 75, 76, 79
self-identity 81, 94, 139, 141
self-reflection 154–5, 156
self-reflexivity 137, 138, **147**, 211
self-worth **93**, 96, 104, 148; CEL and 182, 188, 192; IEL and 162; TEL and 148, 152, 153
shame-anger spirals 183, 184, 186, 189
Smith, P. 31, 32, 41, 44, 155, 169, 172, 207
social constructionist school 51
social hierarchies 41–2
social identity 92, 94, 97, 106, 207; feeling rules 207; and links to CEL 182, 183, 184
social interaction 70–1, 74–5, 85, 87, 98, 203
social order **93**, 96–9, 113, 162, 189, 204, 209
social recognition 94
social status 25–6, 42
social theory of emotion, Hochschild,s new 51, 62–4, 68, 71–80, 86–7
sociology of emotion 26, 51, 87
speed-up: in the airline industry 22–3; in nursing 24, 44–6
Spilius, E.B. 140, 203
spontaneous emotion 83
Stanislavski, Constantin 18
status: clinical skills 44, 206; feeling rules and issues of 205–7; nurse-patient relationship 39, 206; nursing 26; social 25–6, 42; in Ward B 132
status markers 132, 182, 183, 189, 213
Stets, J. 51, 53, 58, 60, 93, 202, 203
Stocker, M. 203
Strongman, K.T. 53, 80
subject-object 93, **93**, 94, 105, 162, **163**, 190
subject-subject **93**, 94, 96, 105, **147**, 167, **182**, 187, 188
subjectivism 91
superego 69, 71, 74, 84, 85, 87, 100, 101
suppressed emotion 106–7, 108, 121–2, 194, 195
surface acting 18, 19–20, 23, 32; inauthenticity and self-deception 40, 75, 76; interactive element 77; links to method acting and dramaturgy 73–4; and personal identity 213–14
surgical nursing 161
Symington, N. 139

Taylor, Charles 91
television programmes 30–1, 32
Theodosius, C. 72, 144
theoretical frameworks in data analysis 140–1

theory of gesture 68–9
therapeutic emotional labour (TEL) 143–57, **196**; autonomy and investment of self in 152–4; comparisons with CEL 180–1; comparisons with IEL 172–3; feeling rules **147**, 217; interpersonal skills necessary for 173; marginalisation of 5–6, 47–8, 156, 168–9, 172, 217–19; in nursing 154–7, 172; power and status 206, 217; in 'The Complaint' vignette 142, 147–51, 154–5, 209, 217; time and space to learn the skills 45, 170
time, trajectories of emotions across 92, 98, 110, 124, 209
Tonkin, E. 125
training nurses: and declining importance of emotional labour in 44; mentoring students 123–4, 174–6, 187–8; reintegrating TEL 218; teaching emotional labour 30, 32, 41, 155
transference 139–40, 141, 187, 203, 211, 212
trust and power: in emotional labour 40–3, 48, 113, 217; in the nurse-patient relationship 40, 41, 43, 48, 113, 217
Turner, J. 51, 53, 58, 60, 93, 202, 203

unconscious, the 57, 69, 79, 140; emotions 78, 139, 141, 203; Freud on 83–6, 87, 106, 108, 114, 210; memory 80; omission by Archer 108, 113–14

vignettes 6–7, 133–4, 136
vomiting patient scenario 107; Archer's approach 101, 105–6, 108; Freud's approach 69; Hochschild's approach 105

Walby, S. 167, 181
Ward B 1–5, 125–33; allocation of work 129–31, 132; bullying 126, 128, 129, 132–3; C Bay myth 130–1, 132; cliques 126, 128–9; establishing status on 132; feelings of satisfaction/dissatisfaction 131–2; layout **127**
Wentworth, W. 202, 203, 205
White Collar 14
Williams, Archbishop Rowan 1, 5, 218
Williams, S. 62, 202, 203, 205
Witz, A. 169
women and emotion work/labour 24–5, 212
Wouters, C. 15, 41

Yardley, D. 202, 203, 205

Zajonc, R.B. 58, 68, 93
Zweckrational 161